You may also like:

- *A Family Physician's Life* by Dr. B.C. Rao

  (A collection of writings from the life and practice of a family physician over half a century)

UNTOLD TALES FROM A FAMILY PHYSICIAN'S BAG

Author

Dr. B.C. Rao

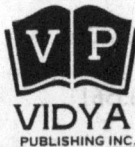

Vidya Publishing Inc.

Toronto Canada Bhubaneswar India

Untold Tales From A Family Physician's Bag
by Dr. B.C. Rao

....

ISBN : 978-1-998475-52-0

First Edition   : March, 2025

Published by   : Dr. Tanmay Panda & Dr. Sunanda Mishra Panda
                     Vidya Publishing Inc.
                     Toronto, Canada || Bhubaneswar, Odisha

Website   : www.vidyapublishing.com
Email   : vidyapublishinginc@gmail.com
Cell   : +1 6478389884

Odisha Contact   : Nirmalya Garden, Plot 516/1719, House 10,
                     KIIT Post Office, Patia, Bhubaneswar - 751024
Cell   : +91 8000455611

Cover Design   : Srushti Panda
                     Printed in India, Biswanath Enterprises

Price   : ₹ 450 /-

Foreword

I feel honoured by Dr. B.C. Rao's request to me to write the foreword to this book. He could easily have chosen someone much better known whose name would then aid in giving the book a higher publicity but he refused to listen to me.

A doctor's profession is undoubtedly the noblest. The early years of my childhood in Calcutta were spent very near the residence of the then Chief Minister of West Bengal, Dr. Bidhan Chandra Roy. B.C. Roy was a doctor par excellence, and every morning, before leaving for office, he saw patients. The treatment was free. The initials of Dr. Rao match those of the legendary Bidhan Chandra Roy. As a doctor he shows the same kind of excellence as Dr. B.C. Roy did in his times.

As Dr. Rao established his practice in Indiranagar more than five decades ago, he discovered that a large number of individuals, who approached him for medical treatment, suffered from one or the other kind of respiratory trouble. My association with him started in 1989 also for the same reason, because I suffered from chronic asthma. Since then he has treated me and later members of my family all these years. Whenever a medical need arose, Dr. Rao was always the 'go to' doctor first and we always felt safe in his hands and followed his advice.

During the years of his practice, he has treated a wide variety of individuals afflicted with as wide a range of diseases. The meticulous notes that he kept of his patients and their ailments have finally impelled him to pen his experiences in two wonderful books – *A Family Physician's Life* (published last year), and now *Untold Tales From A Family Physician's Bag*. By reading the stories we not only get to know of the behavioural aspects of patients and the various diseases, we also learn the technical descriptions of the diseases, some common and some not so common. On the surface, the stories may appear to be funny, but at depth there is always a touch of seriousness, and they always carry subtle messages. A great quality of his storytelling is that he is never harsh and even his displeasure is tempered by his humane approach.

A defining quality of Dr. Rao's personality is his integrity, and his strong emphasis on medical ethics. This quality is rather rare among the practising doctors today.

Dr. Rao has many other interests outside of his profession. He loves playing badminton, and considers it to be a game where all the body muscles are used at their best. He plays golf, which he considers a meditative game, and he loves cricket.

In addition, he is an avid birdwatcher, and a connoisseur of Hindustani Classical Music. *Untold Tales* tells the story of his association with well-known cricketers, musicians and eminent people of other professions.

The book discusses some serious socio-economic issues. We know the decrepit state of government hospitals and how they are avoided by most urban people and thus serve only the poorer sections of the society. The private hospitals are more like commercial establishments managed at the top by trained business executives. Many of them lack the care one finds in a family doctor's service. They also burn a hole in the pocket by almost always recommending a series of tests, many of which may turn out to be quite unnecessary. As Dr. Rao says, given this scenario, there is a great need today for family physicians but doctors rarely take up this activity as a profession.

This *Foreword* is written from the perspective of a patient, and I guess that will prove to be common with most of the readership of the book when it is published. I do hope the readers will appreciate the qualities of a truly great doctor and enjoy savouring his real-life tales.

Dipankar C.V. Mallik,
Astronomer and Author,
Bangalore.

About the Book

Dr. B.C. Rao's *Untold Tales From A Family Physician's Bag* is a captivating collection of anecdotes that offers a unique glimpse into the life and practice of a dedicated family physician. This book beautifully captures the essence of family medicine, intertwining professional challenges, patient interactions, and personal reflections to create a compelling narrative.

Each story is a testament to the profound relationships and trust that define the doctor-patient bond. From humorous and heartwarming to occasionally bittersweet, these tales are steeped in the wisdom and humanity that only decades of experience in family medicine can provide. The stories bring to life not only the author's clinical acumen but also his deep empathy and understanding of the human condition.

Dr. Rao's ability to weave life lessons into everyday encounters makes this book resonate with readers from all walks of life. It reminds us of the invaluable role of the family doctor—not just as a healer but as a confidant, guide, and friend. The author's courageous reflections on contemporary healthcare issues provide a thought-provoking commentary, adding depth and relevance to the evolving landscape of medicine.

This compilation is an inspiring tribute to the *art* of general practice and the enduring value of compassionate care. This is a must-read for medical professionals, aspiring doctors, and anyone who appreciates the intricate tapestry of life's stories as seen through the lens of a family doctor. Dr. Rao's work is both a celebration of the profession and a legacy for generations to come.

Col. [Dr.] Mohan Kubendra,
National President,
Academy of Family Physicians of India [AFPI].

Preface by the Author

I have had the privilege of being a family doctor for over fifty-five years. This book tells stories of my relationships with patients and their families. Notes kept over this period have helped me recall and construct these narratives. I have titled this book *Untold Tales From A Family Physician's Bag* as some have already been told in my earlier book and these in this book have remained to be told.

Some stories and essays are not directly related to health but focus on personalities and my hobbies, such as sports, music, and plant and birdlife.

Medicine has changed considerably in these five decades, with spectacular progress in curative medicine. However, the same cannot be said for preventive medicine and other health-related aspects, such as primary care, its delivery to those in need, and nutrition.

Many stories highlight this aspect of health. Some also reflect the results of aggressive marketing of curative health and how medical education, both undergraduate and postgraduate, is increasingly veering towards institution-based curative health, neglecting primary care and family medicine.

The result is there for all to see: a rampant incidence of preventable illnesses such as diabetes, heart disease, hypertension and obesity, along with late recognition of all types of cancer and the persistence of infections like viral infections, typhoid, malaria, and tuberculosis.

Some stories also illustrate the dilemma of the conflict between curative medicine and primary care, rather than their being complementary.

Three individuals were directly involved in this venture: Durba Biswas, Dipankar C Vasu Mallik, and Swetha Reddy Pitchela. Many thanks to them.

I am also grateful to Dipankar C Vasu Mallik for his foreword and Col. [Dr.] Mohan Kubendra for his comments.

I thank Drs. Sunanda Mishra Panda and Tanmay Panda of Vidya Publishers for their note and for publishing this book in such excellent form.

Many others were indirectly involved, including Kalpna Kar, Swathi Reddy, Prashant Sankaran, and my wife, Vasantha. I apologise if I have inadvertently missed anyone.

I am also grateful to the many readers of my first book and to my patients, who encouraged me to write this second one.

Dr. B.C. Rao [Dr. Badakere Chidambar Rao],
Email: badakere.rao@gmail.com,
Bangalore.

Editorial Notes

As a child, I heard a story from my father about how in Japan, an old villager once could apprehend the coming disaster from the stillness of the sea and the receding waves. The old man had never experienced such a disaster, but he had heard about it from his elders and they from their elders. For generations, the story was passed on by word of mouth. So, when this old man saw the receding waves, he warned the villagers and convinced them to rush to a nearby hilltop. He thus saved the entire village from what we now know as the tsunami. That's the power of stories, the years of knowledge and priceless experience they carry.

Dr. B.C. Rao's chronicles covering his five decades of professional journey as a family physician are a must-read not just for the medical community but also for society at large – these are stories we can easily relate to and learn from. His stories about his patients and their families highlight the role of a family physician and the human values central to the doctor-patient relationship.

His reflections and reminiscences of the various people he came to know and interact with, from the famous Astrophysicist Dr. Vainu Bappu to cricketers like Roger Binny and Gundappa Vishwanath, show us a different side to these remarkable personalities. His articles on birds and their habitats, and the changes in today's world – some good and some not so good – tell us about his deep love for the avian world and his varied interests other than practising medicine – be it social or political.

Lastly, his perfect Victorian English and subtle sense of humour make reading these stories all the more interesting and thoroughly enjoyable!

My family and I have been Dr. B.C. Rao's patients for more than three decades. I don't think I could have navigated through my multiple health issues without him by my side. To date, I have never 'Googled' any of the medical challenges I have had – never has there been a need as I have him as my saviour!

I feel privileged to have had this chance to work on the book with him and am sure that you all will not only benefit from the knowledge embedded across the stories but also thoroughly enjoy reading them.

Durba Biswas,
Former Senior Consultant,
Tata Consultancy Services [TCS].

Editorial Notes

Working alongside Dr. [Capt.] B.C. Rao on *Untold Tales From A Family Physician's Bag* has been a distinct honour and a pure delight.

This unique collection offers a truly captivating voice in contemporary storytelling. The prose blends the elegance of Victorian English with a comfortable, colloquial tone. This distinctive style, combined with Dr. Rao's remarkable ability to vividly depict scenes, immediately draws the reader into each narrative.

These recollections afford readers a privileged glimpse into his consulting room, where they witness vulnerability, strength, and resilience often punctuated by unexpected humour, evincing a humane medical practice blending ethical principles, sharp medical acumen, and his characteristic warmth and grace.

Beyond the consulting room, this collection explores Dr. Rao's diverse interests, from the natural world and the arts (including music and literature) to sports and the complexities of modern society, reflecting his multifaceted personality.

Witnessing firsthand how unique anecdotes, spun from personal encounters, grant a form of literary immortality and ensure the legacies of notable individuals endure has been gratifying (and, let's be honest, a lot of fun!).

Our family's relationship with Dr. Rao extends far beyond the professional; for many decades, he's been a valued part of our lives apart from being our trusted physician.

Healing, humanity, humour, hardships, hope, hobbies, heartfelt hypotheses, high-profile handshakes, heroic hearts—these are the threads Dr. Rao weaves into tales, illustrating a life well-lived and the essential human connection our world needs.

This work is certain to strike a chord with a broad audience, particularly those who cherish the unique tapestry of Bangalore.

Swetha Reddy Pitchela,
Master Technologist,
Hewlett-Packard Enterprise [HPE].

Publisher's Notes

At Vidya Publishing, we believe in the profound impact storytelling has on our understanding of the human experience. It is with great pride and excitement that we present *Untold Tales From A Family Physician's Bag* by Dr. B.C. Rao. In this mesmerising collection, Dr. Rao draws upon his extensive experience as a family physician, sharing poignant anecdotes and insightful reflections that illuminate the often-overlooked human aspects of everyday medical practice.

In today's fast-paced world, we frequently encounter clinical efficiency and technological advancements, yet we often lose sight of the fundamental human connections that underpin the art of medicine. Dr. Rao's narratives serve as a powerful reminder of the compassion, empathy, and resilience at the heart of healthcare. Through his eyes, readers are invited to journey beyond charts and diagnoses into the rich tapestry of human stories—stories of hope, triumph, and at times heart-wrenching loss.

Each chapter is imbued with authenticity and emotional depth, allowing readers to connect with the lives and challenges of patients in ways that statistics and medical jargon cannot. Dr. Rao's ability to weave together personal experiences with broader themes such as love, fear, and healing showcases not only his skill as a writer but also his dedication to the principles of medicine.

This book is not just for medical professionals but for anyone who seeks to understand the intricate dynamics of health and humanity. It serves as a bridge connecting the clinical with the personal, offering valuable lessons that resonate across disciplines. We hope it inspires, informs, and touches the hearts of all who read it.

We extend our heartfelt gratitude to Dr. B.C. Rao for sharing his stories that emerge from compassionate medical practice. Enjoy the journey.

Dr. Sunanda Mishra Panda,
Dr. Tanmay Panda,
Vidya Publishing Inc.

Many thanks to my wife

Dr. B. VASANTHA

*for all the sacrifices she has made in the
course of this long journey.*

TABLE OF CONTENTS

23

1

PATIENTS AS PEOPLE

A Sweet Victory

Diabetes is one of the most eminently preventable disorders. This disorder has now become a money-spinner for pharma companies, diet counsellors, endocrinologists and a special breed of doctors who call themselves diabetologists. There is so much hype built up that this is considered a deadly disease. News, social and electronic media are replete with reports, one way or the other related to this illness, to the extent that India now has the dubious distinction of being known as the diabetes capital of the world.

And our super doctor endocrinologists, taking the cue, repeat this sentence *ad nauseam* in every CME [Continuing Medical Education] that is held on this subject.

One of my patients - let me give him a name, Banwari Lal.

Banwari came to see me some time back. I could see him very anxious and tense.

He said, "Doctor *Saab*, I am going to die."

Banwari is a second-generation patient of mine, and I have known him almost since he was born. Now this strapping forty-plus man who has been healthy so far, is now here, announcing his imminent death.

I asked him, "How are you going to die?"

"Sugar disease," he said with all seriousness.

"How do you know you have one?" I asked.

The story unfolded. Banwari got a phone call a couple of weeks back. The caller identified himself as an executive from Estocare, a nationally known diagnostic company, and he had a great offer, especially suited for successful business leaders.

Our Banwari was suitably impressed with him being amongst this chosen elite and asked what these tests were and the cost. The executive explained that the offer was for forty-five tests and the cost was only 2,000 rupees which otherwise would cost 3,500 rupees. Moreover, their technician would come to Banwari's residence to take the blood sample.

Greatly impressed, Banwari placed the order, and the next day a sample of blood was collected.

The results came by email and amongst these mostly unnecessary tests, there were some marked in bold font suggesting abnormality. Based on his knowledge of sugar disease [his father too has it], Banwari knew that his sugar levels were high and that he, like his father, has this dreaded disorder.

Things would have been different had he come to me in the first place soon after he got the report.

An avid TV watcher, he had heard a discussion on diabetes by a panel of doctors, and he thought it best to consult a clinic solely devoted to this disease. He made an appointment at this super-speciality diabetes clinic and went there accompanied by his wife, on an empty stomach as suggested.

There, his blood was drawn once again, and he was given a breakfast of the clinic's choice. This done, he was asked to get an ECG [Electrocardiogram] and ultrasound of the abdomen done.

When asked why these additional tests, he was told by a nurse who had a permanently fixed smile that it was to find out if he had any additional disease. Thus, held captive in that clinic, Banwari was kept busy till noon when his turn came to see the diabetes specialist doctor. The conversation went along the following lines:

The doctor gravely looked at the open file in front of him and asked, "You are Banwari Lal?"

Banwari confirmed indeed he was.

"You have a problem," said the specialist.

As he already knew this because of the bold font figures, Banwari chose to remain quiet.

"You heard what I said?" asked the specialist. This time Banwari was forced to say yes.

"Your blood sugar and lipids are high, and unless these are brought to normal, you run the risk of complications involving your heart, brain and kidneys which may result in serious complications including death." announced the specialist.

Banwari did know about diabetes, but this disconcerting information about causing death was new to him, as his seventy-five-year-old father is a diabetic and is still alive.

"You need to change your lifestyle, exercise regularly and take medication which I will prescribe now," said the specialist. He proceeded to give a prescription for three types of medications.

Banwari was now asked to go to another room, where sat a lady who specialised in giving advice on diet to diabetics. The lady took his weight and found him overweight by 5 kg.

Banwari is a Guajarati and a devout Jain. The dietary discussion with this lady from Banwari's point of view was very painful.

29

When she learnt that being a Jain his last meal was before sunset, she told him in no uncertain terms that he will have to eat according to her chart and not starve. Banwari telling her that he was not starving fell on deaf ears.

Banwari and his wife were given an hour's talk on each ingredient of the food [displayed on a large tray] that they have and the calorie value of each.

By then it was nearing 2 pm, well past their lunchtime, and in addition to hunger, Banwari also had a headache with all this detailed information stuffed into his head. Banwari's brain finds it difficult to understand information other than what is needed for his business, and this calorie *gilorie* stuff that the diet expert told him was beyond his comprehension, and therefore the headache.

His wife Sunitha too is my patient, and it was she who advised him to see me before he did anything like starting the medication and trying the diet.

Before I saw his reports, I checked his blood pressure and heart. Both were normal, and he had good circulation in the limbs. There was no evidence of any skin fungus. Weight was borderline high. I felt he was in good health.

I opened his file, which had become bulky by now. His fasting sugar was 140 and after food, it was 210. His low-density cholesterol was 140 and triglyceride was 240.

I felt like laughing. He must have seen the expression. He asked, "Doctor *Saab*, why are you laughing?"

I said, "It is a smile of pleasure after seeing these reports; you can get back to normal within the next two months if you follow my advice."

"Then, what about heart attack? kidney attack?" he asked.

"Nothing will happen, and you are not going to die and will outlive your father," I said half in jest.

"But what about my evening meal?" he asked with some anxiety.

"You can have your evening meal before sunset," I replied. I gave him a diet and exercise schedule which would not greatly disturb his lifestyle.

He came back the other day. His fasting sugar was 130 and after food it was 160, and both the low-density cholesterol and triglyceride levels had dropped, and he was on no drugs. I told him to continue the slightly altered lifestyle [a bit more exercise and controlled eating] and assured him that at the next visit, in three months, all the values would be normal.

A very happy and relieved Banwari took a grateful leave, leaving behind a box of sweets.

Hopefully, his gift won't make *me* a diabetic.

❖❖◆❖

Two Friends

Two strapping young men came to my clinic one morning. They introduced themselves as Pemmiah and Kushalappa. I have a soft corner for Kodavas in general, and those from the army in particular. Kushalappa, formerly a Naik, was now a Havildar in a well-known infantry battalion. I could make that out even before he told me that he was from the army by the way he stood and from his haircut, typical of the army.

The other fellow, Pemmiah had his right forefinger stuck in a lemon. Now I knew why these two had come. A finger stuck inside a lemon is a way of treating finger infections and relieving pain. That it does neither is a different matter.

As I had not seen the two of them before, I asked who had sent them to me. The army man said, "John Peter sir." Now, this John Peter and his family were my patients but how this pair knew him, I asked. Pat came the answer. Hockey. These

31

two youngsters, when in school, were coached by this Peter and they were still in touch with their coach. I was really impressed. Although I knew Peter was a sports teacher, I didn't know he had such a positive influence on his past students that they would seek his advice on where to get medical help.

Now comes the real drama.

Pemmiah reluctantly freed his finger from the lemon, and I could see that he had what is called Paronychia [infection of the fingertip extending onto the nail bed]. A common condition one sees in practice. This was ripe for a minor surgical procedure that involved giving an injection of locally acting anaesthetic to the base of the digit on either side and draining the pus, and sometimes partial or full excision of the nail. I explained this to him. Like most patients, Pemmiah too asked if I could give him medicines and avoid the cutting. I said it had to be done and why.

Now the army man intervened and said, "Sir, he appears strong but he is very weak, cannot tolerate even simple pain. He cries even if a mosquito bites him." A highly exaggerated version of his friend's poor pain tolerance.

So, poor Pemmiah had no alternative but to agree. I proceeded to inject the anaesthetic and no sooner I did, Pemmiah's pain disappeared.

He said, "*Saar*, magic, pain gone *Saar*, can I now go home?"

I told him "It will come back in two hours; this injection is given so that you will not have pain when I am removing the infected matter." I got the instruments and dressing materials ready and began to cut the dead skin and incise the ripe abscess. The pus and dark congealed blood spurted out of the incision.

At this time, I heard a thud and the tumbling sound of a chair. Turning around I saw the brave soldier, Kushalappa on the ground, apparently lifeless. On his forehead, there was a deep cut as a result of his fall onto the chair on which he was sitting. Instead of sitting quietly, he had stood up to see the operation proceedings and the sight of blood had made him swoon and fall onto the floor, hitting his forehead on the metal chair's edge on the way down.

Seeing his friend on the ground, Pemmiah, now pain-free, started to sit up on the table. I forcibly pushed him down and asked him to be quiet. I was now faced with the problem of whom to attend to.

I decided to tackle the patient on the floor first. His pulse was okay, and he had started moving his legs. His heartbeat was well-heard, though his blood pressure was low. All these were typical signs of syncope [a kind of swoon] which happens with some people at the sight of blood and gore.

Now it was Pemmiah's turn. He asked me, "*Saar*, why did my friend fall?"

I was in no mood to explain. After I drained his abscess and partially removed his nail, I dressed his wound and, after bandaging his finger, told him to lie down for a while and then get up slowly.

"Why *Saar*, I am not like him, I will not have *chakkar pakkar* [meaning feeling giddy]. See." So saying, he got up and helped me to prop up now-recovering Kushalappa onto the chair.

Now I had time to examine the soldier's wound. The cut was deep and needed to be sutured. The soldier readily agreed. I told him I would do it only on one condition: he should keep his eyes closed until I finished. He agreed and I put him on the table.

"*Saar*, can I see?" - This was from Pemmiah.

Saying a firm no, I made him wait outside in the waiting area so that he was well away from the scene of action. I did not want him also to swoon and fall like his friend.

Kushalappa was indeed a brave soldier. There wasn't a whimper from him when I was injecting the local anaesthetic or afterwards when I was applying the sutures. After the procedure, I asked him to slowly get up. He said, "Sir, you don't worry, I will not fall down." True to his word he did not.

Both made a good recovery.

I wondered, being an infantryman, how Kushalappa would manage if he were to be sent to the battlefront.

❖❖◆❖

The Misunderstood Meal Plan

In the area where I once practised, a large number of Muslims lived [and still do], and in many places they were a majority. One family I recall with mixed feelings was that of Usman Khan. At the time this incident happened, some thirty-odd years back, he must have been in his late forties. A towering person of six feet plus, all muscle and fat, he became my patient, by accident.

He ran a fruit shop in the Shivajinagar market, which I used to frequent for fruit shopping. For some reason, I started going only to his cubicle, and he must have noticed. In the course of time, we became a sort of friends. I also came to know that his shop was just a front and he did the wholesale business of sourcing the produce and distributing it. After he learnt that I was a doctor and practised not far from where he lived, he and his family became my patients.

Usman's late father was a diabetic, and Usman wanted to know if he too had it, as he had lost some weight and was a bit under the weather. His normal weight of 110 kg was now down to 105 kg!

I did a blood test and found his blood sugar was 300 mg/dL [way above normal]. He also had a marginal rise in his blood pressure.

I assured him that with some dieting plus regulated exercise and medicines, he should soon return to normal. Though a bit upset at the turn of events, he was philosophical in accepting his fate. He said, "We inherit a lot of good things from parents, but also some bad things like blood pressure and diabetes."

I told him to come with his wife, Rehana. He was a bit surprised and asked, "Why Rehana?"

I said, "Rehana, because she is the one who cooks food, and she must know what and how much you should eat and when." A bit crestfallen that he needed to take his wife into confidence, he agreed.

Both came to the clinic one morning.

Counselling diabetics on dietary change is one of the jobs I intensely dislike. All of us in various degrees, enjoy eating. A person with diabetes must forego the luxury of eating whatever he wants and whenever he wants. When I start with the common refrain of not eating sweets, avoiding fried food, and eating plenty of vegetables, I could see the expression on their faces changing for the worse.

It is like a life-long death sentence [in most cases, it is true]. I have had a couple of patients who stopped me mid-way and told me in no uncertain terms that they simply could not follow what they considered a starvation diet. One of them, when I was telling him to eat no more than three small *idlis* [steamed cakes made from a fermented rice and lentil batter] for breakfast, told me that he eats all fifteen idlis cooked by the house idli-maker [a device with three trays, each holding five portions of batter]. My suggestion that he eat only three must have come as a great shock to him. No wonder he stopped me from continuing.

Now coming back to Usman and Rehana. I began with the need to exercise.

I asked Usman, "What is the exercise you are doing now?"

He said, "I walk to the shop and back, Doctor *Saab*."

"He is not telling the truth [*eh jhute bolthe hain*, in Urdu]; he goes on a motorbike, and only rarely he goes by walk," said Rehana.

One of my doctor friends had once told me that if you want to know the truth, ask the wife.

Rehana got a glare from Usman for revealing the truth.

I began explaining why he must not only walk to the shop, which was just a couple of kilometres away, but also walk for an hour daily, and I explained the proper pace for such a walk. I also told him if he could walk for one hour in the evening, it would do him a world of good.

He was silent but Rehana was not. She said, "Doctor *Saab*, how will he walk in the evening? He comes home only by 9 pm, eats, and sleeps. I have told him one hundred times to come home early, will he ever listen?"

This resulted in Usman giving her another glare.

Now I proceeded to discuss diet, the painful part of the whole process. With many interjections and criticisms from his wife regarding his irregular eating habits and his love for sweets and fried food, the consultation was at last over, with an assurance from Usman that he would try his best.

He came a month later, this time without his wife. His blood sugar was slightly less but still out of control. He said that since he had begun walking and limiting his sweet intake, he was feeling better. I made some adjustments to his medication and sent him home.

One morning Usman called me and said, "My son Siraj has a fever; he is too ill to be brought to the clinic; will you please do a house call before you start work?" He gave me directions to his house, which were easy enough, as I had visited his neighbour's house in the past.

For some reason, I could not do the house call till late in the afternoon, and when I did go there, it was nearing 2 pm. I went into the house to a warm welcome from Rehana and found Usman just preparing to have his lunch. On his plate, I found a large helping of mutton curry and a thick *paratha* [layered whole wheat flatbread], which had nearly filled his plate.

I asked him, "How many of these do you eat?"

He said, "Only two as you told me to."

I had told him two *rotis* and had not specified the girth or the dimensions and he has been following my instruction of two rotis faithfully. Those two rotis/parathas could easily be six small dry rotis I had in my mind when I was counselling them!

As my job was first to see his ill son, I went to see the boy. He was already feeling better since morning having taken a paracetamol tablet.

"Doctor *Saab*, I know you don't eat meat, at least have a bowl of *kheer* [liquid sweet made of vermicelli]," Usman requested.

Not only did my friend eat two large parathas, but he also topped it off with a bowl of this sweet. I couldn't help but show my displeasure at him not following my advice.

"Doctor *Saab*, he ate four parathas and the sweet in a bigger bowl before he started dieting," Rehana said adding insult to injury.

Both listened to my renewed sermon in silence and assured me of better compliance in the future. That it did not happen entirely to my liking is another matter.

The family remained my patients for a long time and despite poor control, Usman lived to be seventy and died of causes other than diabetes.

❖❖◆❖❖

The Endless Complaints Clinic

These days, as I grow older [also wiser?], I am reluctant to take on new patients and the added responsibility. The main reason is that I have come to value my private time much more than before. Another reason is the fear that I may not be able to give an efficient service by my own standards. Be that as it may, I still must take a few because of many compulsions. One such is my own friends who bring their near and dear ones, and I owe it to them, so I accept. Here is one such patient.

This old lady walks in and tells me that she is a very good friend of Mr. G, and because of his recommendation, she has come to see me.

"You look good," she said, opening the consultation. I am used to patients telling me their complaints but not complimenting me on my looks. I sat looking at her, rather confused, and did not know how to respond. She must have guessed and said, "You don't know how to take a compliment." This is true; it leaves me uncomfortable because I suspect the motive, which I know is not the right thing to do.

I said a belated thanks and asked her what I could do for her.

She sat thinking. A few minutes passed.

I asked her again what her reason was for coming to see me. "Oh, that is because Mr. G told me to see you," she said.

We were now back to square one. Many of us, old persons, are forgetful and I thought this one must be one of those. So, I asked her, "Have you forgotten why you are here?"

"Come on doctor, I am not that old. I remember all my problems, the trouble is that there are so many of them, I don't know where to begin."

This was enough to make my heart sink.

I asked her, "What is your problem?"

She began her complaints with *unusual* gusto.

"Thirty years ago, I was involved in an accident and since then I have this periodic headache." She went on to give a graphic description of how the accident took place, the number of doctors she had seen, the investigations that had been done, the medications she was presently on, and the diet she had been following.

Seeing me getting ready to examine her, she said, "Hold on, I also have diabetes and high blood pressure." She proceeded to give another lengthy description.

Then came the description of her knee joint pains. Then her gas in the belly.

There was a brief intermission when she was collecting her thoughts as to her next problem.

"Ha, I also have this ache in my back and pricking sensations in my legs. Sometimes I get up too often at night and this disturbs my husband." A description of how irritable her husband was followed.

You may think that I sat there docile without interrupting her. My attempts were firmly put down with, "Wait a second, I will come to that," or some such comment to keep me in my place.

At last, after nearly half an hour, she allowed me to examine her. There was not much wrong with her. I was able to reduce her medications from the twelve drugs to six essential ones. I thought she would be happy. Instead, she said, "But, Doc, I have been taking these for over ten years." A mild argument as to the need to cut down unnecessary medication ensued. She reluctantly agreed to do so.

By now, I was feeling the beginning of a small ache in my head and was having visions of my mid-morning tea.

"When should I come back?" she asked.

"*Six months* from now." I said.

She was taken aback. "But my doctor sees me every month."

I said, "See him every month, but see me once in six months."

She gave a strange look, thanked me, and went away.

I heaved a sigh of relief that I would not have to see her for another six months.

❖❖❖❖

Specialist Treatment

When Mohammed Saifuddin and his family became my patients, some forty-five years ago, I had been in practice for about ten years and was just establishing myself. For a while, I was not his first choice; he came to see me only when his own doctor was unavailable, when his clinic was too busy, or when his treatments did not work. Later, he chose me because I was easy to see, and my clinic was generally not overcrowded.

40

Saifuddin had just retired from service and settled in the newly developing extension with his wife and his eldest son Sulthan's family. They lived nearby, and my clinic was easily accessible. Saifuddin was an impressive, big-built man with a goatee, always in spotless white clothing, and usually came with some complaint concerning his wife or son. In the course of time, I came to call him Mia.

One day, he came to see me. One look at him and I could see that there was some worry bugging him.

I asked him, "What is the problem, Mia?"

"This BP [blood pressure] *beemari* [illness] has struck me," he said.

I asked him, "How do you know?"

He replied, "My doctor niece, Hafeeza, checked and told me."

"Some rise in the BP in your age is not uncommon and easy to treat," I said.

That seemed to mollify him a bit, but still, he said, "My niece told me that I will get a stroke because of this high BP."

Instead of arguing to the contrary, I made him lie down and examined him. He was fit except for the borderline high BP. I told him so.

"With very little medication, your BP will become normal and your chances of getting a stroke will be like in anybody's case. But you need to get some basic tests done." I proceeded to give him a note for blood and urine tests.

He came back a couple of days later with the reports, and they were all normal. His blood pressure was also under control with an alternate-day dose of the mild drug that I had prescribed.

I thought he went home satisfied. But he was not. The BP bug had taken over his thinking. He came back a week later.

41

He had a BP recording machine with him. Unlike the present-day elegant electronic machines, those days we had to rely on the mercury ones and this he had bought.

I asked him, "Mia, why did you buy this?"

"Because you asked me to come every fortnight for a check-up, I thought of checking at home and see you only if it goes high."

This argument had some merit. I proceeded to teach him and his son how to take the measurements using a stethoscope.

While taking leave, he asked me, "How did I get this *shaithan beemari* [demon disease]?"

I tried to tell him it was not so, but he was not impressed. His niece, who had just become a doctor must have impressed him more than me, with all the possible complications of high BP she had recently learnt from her medical college days!

Mia would come now and then to get the BP checked and compare the reading with his home recordings. Given his anxious nature, the blood pressure reading taken in the clinic was always higher than one taken at home.

A worried Mia came one morning, with the chart of BP readings done over the last fifteen days. Most were within the range, but a few were outside the normal range. He asked me, "Why my BP is like this? One day high and one day normal?"

I tried explaining, "Mia, it is like this; BP is variable and changes depending on your mental and physical activity. In your case, it is mostly normal but once in a while, it is slightly above normal. You should not worry and do not take the BP daily, that itself will become a disease."

Appearing reassured, he went his way.

He saw me again six months later. What was he doing in these six months?

42

Those days, the city was comparatively small and there were very few specialists. One such specialist was Dr. Parashuram. This foreign-qualified specialist was a *character*. Nowadays you see a photo of a specialist, working in this hospital or doing this surgery or procedure and saving lives, *etc.*, appearing in print and electronic media and gaining much-needed publicity and thereby patients.

Unlike today, Parashuram's name didn't appear in the media directly, but he had plenty of indirect publicity. Not a week passed without his name appearing in the daily newspapers, that he had attended to a sick minister or given a lecture in some meeting or the other. He also had excellent manners which impressed people who met him.

I too had an experience of meeting him and though not very impressed with his knowledge, was impressed with his way with patients.

Our Mia, very unwell, due to the *khatharnak* [very dangerous] disease of BP, came to know about this *mister cure-all* specialist and decided to visit him. So, on an afternoon, Mia, dressed to kill, went with his son to see this Dr. Parasram [pronounced thus by him]. At the entrance of the building, a watchman stopped the father and son duo and asked them why they were there.

Our Mia thought he was asking for their names, and said, "I am Mohammed Saifuddin, and this is my son, Sulthan."

The irritated guard said, "I did not ask your names, I wanted to know why you are here."

Mia said, "To see the doctor."

The security guard directed them to the doctor's chambers, located some distance away among other similar offices.

Here they were greeted to a spectacle of some twenty patients and relatives sitting in a large room with a lady behind a desk manning a phone and appearing very busy. Sulthan and Mia were impressed with this display of waiting patients, the well-appointed waiting area, and the busy lady behind the high desk. They had to wait for a while for the lady to finish her talk.

She asked, "Have you come to see the doctor?" Mia said, "Yes."

Then she asked, "Do you have an appointment?"

This was new. The pair had thought they could see the doctor immediately or after some wait as they did when they came to see me.

They said that they did not have an appointment. The lady added after referring to her book, "You can see the doctor after ten days at 3 pm," and without giving any chance for them to speak, she took down their names and phone numbers and requested them to be on time that day.

So, saying, she dismissed them.

Instead of getting put-off by this, Mia and to some extent the son Sulthan were very impressed.

Mia thought that if there was one doctor in the city who could cure him of this blessed BP, it was this Parasram. So thinking, he and Sulthan returned home.

On the given day, they were there on time at 3 pm. Some patients were already waiting, but there was no sign of the doctor. When they went and asked the now idling receptionist, she told them, "He is busy in the hospital; it will be an hour before he comes; after that, you will be fourth, after those three," and pointed her shapely finger at the waiting patients. So, they waited.

Dr. Parasram arrived an hour and a half later, and it was nearly 6 pm when Mia's turn came to see the doctor. Mia looked at the doctor and the well-decorated room with one

44

side displaying all the earned and unearned degrees and citations received by the doctor and the large, polished desk adorned by two phones and the person of Dr. Parasram sitting behind, red-faced, well-built in a blue suit and a ready, welcoming smile on the face. Mia was very impressed. Both the father and son were asked to take their seats, and the conversation went on like this.

"How are you, Mr. Saifuddin?"

To which Saifuddin replied, "Not well, Doctor. I've had this BP problem for six months, and it's not improving despite taking medication."

Did our good Parasram say that BP is not a disease? No such thing. He said, "We will see what can be done."

He made Mia remove his *sherwani* [coat] and vest and lie down on the couch.

Dr. Parasram spent the next ten minutes checking Mia's pulse, BP, and heart, peered into his eyes, and finished his examination. Then looking at Mia he said gravely, "Yes, you have high BP. We need to do some tests to find out if it has affected other organs of your body."

At this, though a bit frightened, Mia was even more impressed.

Dr. Parasram gave a letter listing blood and urine tests, a chest X-ray, and an ECG. As it was late, Mia went to a nearby laboratory the next day and got all the tests done. With the reports, he was asked to come three days later to see the doctor.

This time, the following conversation took place between the doctor and Mia.

The doctor started by saying, "Mr. Saifuddin, you have high BP. Luckily for you, your heart is not damaged though it is a bit bigger than normal due to long-standing untreated blood pressure."

At this, Mia interrupted and said, "But doctor, I am under treatment with this medicine," and cited the name of the medicine.

"But it has not acted well; you need stronger medicine than what your doctor has prescribed; you need to take this and come back after two weeks," Dr. Parasram said and gave a prescription for new drugs.

After two weeks, Mia made another pilgrimage to the city, this time after fixing an appointment. The same story of waiting *etc.* was repeated this time too. As he complained of tension about the impending BP test, the doctor added a tranquiliser pill to the drug list. Mia made this pilgrimage five to six times in the next six months.

After parting with a considerable amount of money in the form of doctor's fees and tests and medicines, going through the rigors of travel and waiting, and finding that his BP was still fluctuating, Mia felt it wise to see his old doctor again.

He thus appeared one day at my clinic. I knew he was seeing this specialist because his son Sulthan had mentioned it during one of his visits to my clinic.

After the usual greetings, I asked him, "Mia, what brings you here?"

"I am tired of going to see Dr. Parasram. He gives different types of *goli* [tablet] each time I visit and does tests, and despite all that my BP still goes up and down, like it did when you were treating me. I am also having this trouble of all the time feeling sleepy."

I had no quick answer and felt it would be better to examine him. I went through all the tests done and the drugs he was taking. The examination was normal, and he was on two types of BP medicines, one type of vitamin and minerals pill, and one tranquiliser pill. The tests done a couple of times were all normal, including his ECG and X-ray.

I spent the next half an hour patiently explaining why the BP fluctuates, why it is ok if it is within the acceptable range, that getting a stroke is only remotely possible, and that his sleepy feeling was due to taking a sleeping pill in the morning and evening. It took some convincing to do away with the vitamin and the sleeping pill and reduce the BP medication.

For the next twenty years, he regularly saw me and passed away at the ripe old age of eighty-five due to a stroke but with his BP all the time being within the normal range.

❖❖❖❖

The Swoon and After
(Written some years back)

I have heard and read stories of people collapsing and even having heart attacks, sometimes resulting in death, when they hear distressing news. In my fifty-odd years of being a doctor, breaking unpleasant news to many of my patients and watching their agony, I had rarely come across anyone who swooned, had a stroke or a heart attack, or died. That is, *until* a week ago.

This fifty-year-old Mrs. P came in with a young man Mr. S. He was a house guest with Mrs. P and would stay with her till he found accommodation. The reason why she brought him was that Mr. S had a fever for the past three days and felt very dizzy the previous night and with difficulty prevented a fall. She made fun of the youngster saying how little resistance the modern youngsters have when compared to people of her age and gave her example of good health and how infrequently she saw doctors.

In fact, she asked me, "When was the last time that you saw me?" I really did not know, and her face was just vaguely familiar. If she had not told me, I would not have thought that she was ever my patient. I told her truthfully that it must have been a long time ago.

"See, what did I tell you?" she said looking accusingly at Mr. S, as if by falling sick he had committed some form of crime.

There was not much wrong with the young man except for lower-than-normal blood pressure which combined with his fever must have caused some momentary dizziness. I reassured him of the nature of the illness, which would probably limit itself, and he should be alright in a couple of days. Mrs. P could not help saying, "I told you it is nothing to worry about, but you would not listen. See, now the doctor also tells you the same." The tone clearly indicated that coming to see me was a waste of time.

She would not leave. "Doctor," she said, "Will you please check my blood pressure also?" This kind of free additional consultation is part of the game and I do not mind doing it these days. I checked her blood pressure, and to my surprise, this *super-fit* woman [her assumption] had high blood pressure. I told her so and told her to get back in the evening for a re-check and made a note for some basic tests before beginning the treatment.

She did not answer. Instead, she said she was feeling giddy. I made her sit in the waiting area and proceeded to see the next patient. A few minutes later, Mr. S came in and said, "Doctor, come and see her; she is not talking."

I went out and found her head had rolled to one side. We laid her down, and she had a fit [convulsed]. Soon after, she opened her eyes and was surprised at finding herself on the floor instead of sitting on the chair. By now, I had again taken her blood pressure, which had dropped to near-normal levels. Heart rate and rhythm were normal, and she seemed to be fine. She wanted to go home having profusely apologised for *creating a scene*.

48

I would not let her. A person with high BP who swoons and has an observed fit and blood pressure drop could have had a heart attack, a stroke, or even a tumour in her brain for all one knows. I explained why she must go to a hospital. My suggestion that I call an ambulance was vetoed by her. By now, she had recovered well enough to call a friend to come over and take her to the hospital. The friend duly arrived, and the now-recovered lady was slowly moved to the car and taken away.

The drama took over an hour of my time. I went back to work. After half an hour Mr. S came in and asked, "Doctor, do you know where Mrs. P lives? They have left me here and have gone to the hospital. I do not have her phone number or her address. I do not know how to go back!"

Now I was faced with a new problem. How to get this man home? I did not know where Mrs. P lived, except somewhere nearby. I told him that he had the options of sitting in the waiting room until Mrs. P and her companion realised that they had left him behind or going over to the hospital and finding them. This poor man's face fell, faced with this daunting task. He quietly returned to the waiting area.

I went out an hour later and found that he had gone.

The consultant from the hospital called to say that the lady's blood pressure was normal, her ECG was also normal, and they are waiting for the brain scan reports. Mrs. P came to see me with all the reports after a week. All were normal. It only confirmed that what she had was indeed a syncopal fit on hearing the bad news!

She reluctantly agreed to begin taking medications for her raised blood pressure.

✧✧✦✧✧

Deaf and Dumb Narayana

People from Coastal Karnataka speak many languages, but principally two: Kannada and Tulu. Most Tulu speakers also speak Kannada, and vice versa. They also intermarry. It may be interesting to know that a small river [Mabukala], which flows from the Western Ghats and joins the Arabian Sea, separates these two groups. Those to the north of the river speak Kannada, and those to the south speak Tulu. The Kannada they speak is a dialect that regular Kannadigas would find difficult to understand. Hailing from this area, I am conversant with this dialect, which I also spoke during my childhood.

These people have one characteristic that distinguishes them from the rest of Karnataka: they are, by birth, a kind of footloose migrants. They migrate to other parts of the state and country, and through their hard work ethic, they succeed in their ventures, as you can see today by the proliferation of eateries called *Darshinis* in Bangalore. One such family chose me as their family doctor precisely because I hailed from this part of the state and understood the lingo.

This happened many years ago. This young and harried mother used to bring her ten-year-old son to see me. The boy was an introvert, performed poorly at school, frequently fell ill, and, to add insult to injury, he was a very poor communicator. The father, Keshu Shetty, was a small eatery owner and had two other sons who met the family's expectations in developing the required social skills and scholastic performance.

They belonged to a reasonably affluent and high-performing family with many wealthy professionals and businessmen and thus suffered by comparison. Therefore, managing this boy, whose full name was Thumbe Narayana Shetty, was stressful for everyone. His mother called him *Gadde* [which means swelling], and I called him *Mooka* [deaf and dumb]. I never

50

asked why his mother called him Gadde but my calling him Mooka had reasons. Whenever a question was asked, his response was a blank stare, as though he had never heard you, and therefore he would not answer.

That he understood and that his hearing was normal was clear by the way he opened his mouth when asked to and his response to my other such requests. But he would not speak and would only grunt. My attempts to humour him also used to fail, and I had never seen him smile in the years that his mother suffered with him, and I saw him. To put it in a nutshell, he had all the makings of the family's forthcoming disaster.

More to humour his mother than the boy, I used to give many examples of such apparently dull children [like Einstein] becoming highly successful scientists and even gave an example of one of my own classmates who couldn't understand the basics of physiology, going on to become one of the most famous nephrologists in the country. But she was rightly sceptical of my optimism.

This community, to which the boy belonged, goes by the clan's name of Bunt. There are many famous Bunts. Our own Dr. Deviprasad Shetty is one, and the famous beauty Aishwarya Rai Bachchan and many Shetty women film stars are others. That the community has also produced several leaders of the underworld is a different matter altogether.

They are a gutsy and handsome people and usually excel in whatever they undertake. Our 'deaf and dumb' Narayana was going to be an exception or so we all thought.

Some months ago, I had a visitor who sent in his driver, who gave me a card and said his boss wanted to see me. The card read "Narayan Keshu Tumbe" and gave a fancy address in Pune. I had to make the gentleman wait for some time, and after I was done with the waiting patients, I asked him to come in. In walked a man in his late forties, class reeking

51

from every pore of his body, and asked me, "How are you, Doctor? You haven't changed much since the time I used to see you."

Seeing my blank expression, he said, "You called me *deaf and dumb* Narayana."

Memories of the 'deaf and dumb' Narayana came flooding back, and looking at this handsome, successful man, I just couldn't believe it was the same boy who now stood so confidently in front of me.

I was curious to know why he had come to see me. He was obviously not ill.

He said, "I just felt like seeing you; you were one of the few persons who believed I would be successful [the stories of Einstein and others I told his mother!]."

I asked him what he had been doing since I last saw him. He said he now owns a chain of bars and restaurants across cities in Maharashtra and jokingly said he had changed his name to sound Maharashtrian!

I asked about his parents. "My father is no more, but my mother is with me," he said. I then asked about his academically bright brothers. "Oh, they both work for me," he said.

He said goodbye, leaving behind a basket of fruit and a huge bouquet of flowers. I went out to see him off. He got into his chauffeur-driven limousine and drove off.

Our *deaf and dumb* Narayana!

❖❖❖❖

Taken for a Ride?
(Written many years back)

Mine is a fee-for-service kind of practice where, after each consultation, the patient pays. There is no fixed fee, and this was truer in the early years of my practice than in the later years. There were many patients who intentionally or otherwise succeeded in making me believe that they were of limited means and thus got away without paying my fee or paying much less than my usual fee. My main difficulty, then, and occasionally now, is to find out the capacity of the patient to pay.

Narayanappa was an infrequent visitor to my clinic. His asthma was mild and seasonal, and like many of my patients, he too self-medicated, often using my old prescriptions, and was none the worse for it. He was another of my many misjudgements. Whenever he came, he would be wrapped in an old, torn *kambal* [blanket], with a dirty muffler around his neck, and wearing his standard off-white pyjamas and *kurta*, which had seen better days. He also came unaccompanied, and I had not met his family members. I came to know that he was very well-off only by sheer accident.

One can make out which part of the country a patient came from by how one dresses, by one's accent, or by one's attitude, but not by one's ability to pay. Sometimes I could make out by the questions they asked. A Keralite would ask me if he could have a bath, as his daily bath is more important than almost anything else in life. A Tamilian would ask me what he should eat and what he should avoid eating. A Kannadiga would ask how much rest he needed and how many days should he take off from work. None of these helped me in assessing their monetary status.

Narayanappa was an unusual Kannadiga, and on one occasion, when he was about to leave, he asked me whether he could drink *kaach*. This had me wondering for a moment

53

before it dawned on me that my seemingly indigent patient was asking me whether he could drink his usual tot of Scotch whisky at night! When his doctor is struggling to have his weekly mug of beer, here was a patient who was asking him whether he could have his daily dose of Scotch whisky.

I did not begrudge him this travesty of justice or his whisky but the many occasions that I took no money from him, thinking that he was too poor to pay! I told him he could drink but refrained from asking for whatever he owed me, as I keep no track of the free service I do.

But next time he came, he paid double my usual fee, and then, until he stopped coming, he paid more than others without a whimper.

❖❖◆❖

The Well-Disguised Wealth
(Written many years back)

He always came accompanied by another young man. This young man first came into the clinic, confirmed that I was available, and after that, they both would come in. He would then dismiss the youngster and ask him to wait outside. He was well past sixty and in reasonable health. He had no major illness except for the age-onset blood pressure. Though there was no real need for him to come every month, and despite my advice that he needed to come only once every three months, he visited me every month.

His dress was always the same. He wore a white shirt and trousers, over which he wore a dark coat. All these were long past their prime. By his mannerisms and looks, I took him to be a retired, rather impoverished schoolteacher. I treated schoolteachers at concessional rates, and this man, too, was treated that way, though often he tried to pay my normal fee, which I politely declined.

54

I took it for granted that the young man was his son and came with his father as a kind of physical and moral support, though the sequence of events, as described here, was unusual in a father-and-son relationship.

The consultation was always brief and to the point. He wasted no time on gossip, would attempt to pay my regular fee, and on my refusal, would thank me with a smile and take his leave.

One day, in the office, I found him talking to a group of people outside, and these appeared important by their mannerisms and the way they were dressed. They apparently had come in search of him, and having found him, were discussing some matter of importance.

After a while, he came in, leaving his 'son' outside. After the consultation was over, I couldn't help asking him about the crowd waiting outside. He said they were traders from Coimbatore who had come to see him. I was intrigued. What did this retired schoolmaster have to do with traders from Coimbatore? I asked him. He guffawed and said, "I grow potatoes and vegetables on my farm, and they come to buy from me."

I sat there looking at this 'poor' man, who, with his extended family, was one of the largest producers of potatoes and vegetables on his family's farm!

The youngster who chaperoned him was his driver and *man Friday*!

Looks can be so deceptive!

The old man is no more, but the members of his extended family continue to be my patients.

❖❖◆❖

55

Art of the Placebo

I have written about family doctors whom I observed while growing up and during the early years of my practice. Dr. Ganapayya was one of them. His daughter, Githa, and I are good friends and medical school classmates. This strengthened the bond that developed between Dr. Ganapayya and me. As luck would have it, when I wanted to open a branch clinic in another area, it happened to be in the same area as Dr. Ganapayya's.

Many facets of practice I learnt by observing him practise and by accompanying him on house calls. He was a short, muscular, bespectacled man, always with a smile on his face, and short-tempered when the occasion demanded. His practice covered a large geographical area, including present-day Banaswadi, Kalkere, Bagalur, Maruthisevanagar, Kammanhalli, Lingarajapuram, Horamavu, Hennur, and other villages located some ten to fifteen kilometres from his core practice area in Cox Town, Fraser Town, Mosque Road, Sindhi Colony, Cleveland Town, Russell Market, and Tannery Road. Some of these names remain, whilst others have changed.

The city of Bangalore has now spread far beyond these villages. Then, some forty years ago, these areas were connected to the city by single-track roads with vineyards on either side, and it was a pleasure to drive and observe the lush fields and surrounding scenery, which is a stark contrast to the present-day *concrete jungle* they have become.

One forenoon, finding no patients waiting for me in my clinic, I went to see Dr. Ganapayya. As he was busy with a patient, I sat in the waiting area. Some more patients were waiting to see him. While waiting, I heard the loud voice of Dr. G shouting at the patient and telling him to get out [in chaste Urdu]. And I saw the patient walking out of the room rubbing his cheek. It was obvious that the doctor had slapped him.

He came and sat by my side still rubbing his cheek. I asked him, "What happened?"

He said, "Doctor *ne thappad mara* [Doctor slapped me]."

I asked him, "Why?"

"I stopped taking medicine," he replied.

"Why did you stop?" I asked.

"My mother-in-law told me English medicine is *kharab* [bad]," he said. "I told this to the doctor, and he got very angry and slapped me." I too probably would have reacted similarly if my patient had followed his mother-in-law's advice instead of mine.

"Now that the doctor has asked you to get out and not come back, what will you do?" I asked.

He said, "I know this doctor, he is like my father. After some time, I will go in. By then he would have cooled down and he will see me."

This was the kind of relationship we doctors had with our patients then. Can you think of such a thing happening *now*?

Another instance involved a Muslim lady who came all the way from Yeshwanthpur, some twenty kilometres away. For this, she had to change buses twice which took nearly two hours. Another hour of waiting to see the doctor and two hours more to get back to her home. Nearly half a day gone. The consultation with the doctor must have taken not even ten minutes.

The conversation began like this in Urdu:

"What is the problem Fathima Beevi, this time?"

"Same as last time Doctor *Saab* [sir]," said Fathima Beevi.

Dr. G felt her pulse, looked at her eyes and throat, placed the stethoscope on her chest, and called out to his compounder,

"Give this lady the *peela davai* [yellow medicine] for one month."

"When should I come back?" Fathima Beevi asked.

"After one month," said the doctor.

"*Meharbani, Shukriya* [thank you]," said Fathima and took her leave after collecting the precious yellow mixture.

Curious to know the secret of this yellow medicine and the nature of her complaint as she had not told her problem to the doctor, I asked Dr. G about it. He said, "'Same problem' means aches in the head, limbs, back, no sleep, racing heart, *etc*. She has been having these for the last five years. She is a very unhappy woman with a lot of family problems, and coming here helps her to get away from these problems for half a day. The *peela davai* a yellow, alkaline mixture is to be taken two spoons daily for a month. She will faithfully take it and come here again for her half a day's outing."

This left me thinking.

Another time, while I was sitting with him, a patient came in with a vial of B12 injection. He received the injection and left. No examination, no discussion: just injection, payment, and departure.

I asked the doctor.

He said, "This patient *swears by* this injection, and he takes it every two weeks. When he first came some three years back, he had some complaints like aches, pins and needles in his limbs, weakness, and other vague symptoms and I gave him a couple of B12 injections for a few weeks. He became so much better that he wants to continue taking this. I have tried telling him that it is not required; he will not listen and insists on taking this. As it does not harm, I give it, and he is happy."

58

Another time I went out on a house call with him to see one of his patients. A school-going girl was sick with a fever. We were late for the house call and the doctor apologised for being late. The lady [girl's mother] was very anxious and wringing her hands in distress she said, "Doctor, Mridula has a very high fever. I have given her aspirin, but her fever is not coming down."

Both of us went in to see this girl with a high fever. She did not look very sick and was in bed reading a comic book. Dr. G spent some time examining her, and told the mother to come to his clinic and collect a bottle of diaphoretic [he used the words *red mixture*] and give it three times a day for the next two days, expecting the girl to recover by then.

As an afterthought he continued, "In the meantime, you give her a glass of water or fruit juice every four hours and keep changing the wet cloth over her forehead every two hours." The mother looked satisfied.

On the way back, I asked him the rationale behind this advice.

He said, "See, that mother, I have known her for a long time. She is a very anxious person and needs to be kept occupied. These four-hourly preparations of fruit juice and the two-hourly changing of cloth pad will keep her busy and her anxiety will lessen."

I learnt another aspect of practice.

It is well-known that patients respond differently to different doctors. Some achieve better responses than others. Their decisions are often based on their training and experience. These decisions need not always benefit patients. Some medications, while not strictly required, do produce desirable results. This is known as the *placebo effect*. This often comes into play in family medical practice.

59

Often a generalist, like a family doctor, scores over an organ specialist because he looks at the problem holistically and broadly and does not confine his attention to a single organ system.

There is also what is known as the *Rashomon effect*, which influences the decisions made by doctors and patients.

❖❖◆❖❖

Dr. Ramaraj's Heart Attack

When he suffered his first heart attack, Dr. Ramaraj was in his late fifties and weighed 105 kg. In addition to gross obesity, he also had high blood pressure and diabetes. Dr. Ramaraj was a foodie and often said that he lived to eat, and he loved his food. He was quite active in the IMA [Indian Medical Association] those days and had a lot of doctor friends. I was also one of them and the story that follows was told to me by him.

One fine evening he was in his clinic when he developed chest discomfort with sweating, and he knew he was heading for a heart attack. He called his wife and told her to meet him in Bangalore Nursing Home [one of the few small, private hospitals then existing in the city], took his car out and went to that hospital located not far from his area of practice. He had also informed Dr. R. Rao, who was his friend and a heart specialist.

Before I describe what happened next to Ramaraj, I must explain the conditions that prevailed forty years back in the city and the way we treated patients who suffered heart attacks.

There was no Echo, no enzyme testing, but just blood pressure, pulse, and ECG recordings. That was all. No stenting, no bypass grafting, no TMT, no primary angioplasty. The treatment was strict bed rest and severe dieting, consisting of bland food. The bed rest was for four weeks and during the first week it was absolute, and the patient passed urine and stool in bed, using a urinal and a bedpan.

The present-day doctors will *laugh at* this, but that was the norm then.

Dr. R duly arrived, and the ECG revealed an inferior wall infarct, a relatively minor heart muscle injury, with no rhythm disturbance. A heart attack is a heart attack, and the treatment is the same. In Ramaraj's case, it involved a severe weight-reducing diet. His pain soon disappeared [due to the effect of pethidine], and another pain started.

Ramaraj was used to three meals a day, plus small eats every now and then. Now he was past his mealtime, and he was having severe hunger pains. His wife was to come with his night meal and he was anxiously waiting for her. After what seemed like ages, she finally arrived with a tiffin carrier.

A very hungry Ramaraj opened the carrier. The top compartment contained pieces of cucumber, tomato, and carrot. The next compartment had some curd, and the last compartment was empty.

An angry and grief-stricken Ramaraj asked his wife, "What is this?"

"This is what your friend Dr. R has permitted me to bring," the dutiful wife replied.

Ramaraj had no answer but to give his wife a baleful stare.

After two days of this vegetable and curd rice punishment, a desperate Ramaraj tried a new ploy.

He called the sweeper woman and asked, "Will you do a small job for me?" with an appealing *"Please."*

"I will try," the lady said.

Ramaraj took out a ten rupee note and told her, "Please bring me four *idlis* and two *vadas* with *sambar* and *chutney*."

The cleaning lady took the money and went.

A hungry Ramaraj waited.

An hour later, the staff nurse came to see Ramaraj, along with the cleaning lady. The cleaning lady had no parcel with her.

The nurse told Ramaraj, "It is against the rules to eat food not prescribed by the doctor. This lady did not know you are on a diet. Now she knows. She has come to return your money."

They left a crestfallen Ramaraj behind.

On the fourth day, he was allowed to have some well-cooked rice with a bowl of curd. There was a gradual improvement in his diet [but not what he wanted], and he was discharged after four weeks. He later told all of us that it was a punishment worse than death.

He lived for another ten years with multiple problems due to chronic heart failure. He regained the lost weight in a record time of three months and added some more in the next few years.

He died peacefully in his sleep.

❖❖◆❖❖

Story of a Bizarre Illness

Suryanarayana was sixty-five years old when I saw him with this problem. He is now seventy-six and in good health.

This was not so when he saw me eleven years back. I have known him since his college days and after retirement from a Bank, he went and settled in a small town called Krishnapura, near the city of Mangalore. After he and his family went and settled in Krishnapura, I sort of lost contact with him and it was therefore a bit of a surprise to see him, especially in such a poor state of health.

He looked very ill, emaciated, and barely able to walk. The skin hung loose all over the body but severely around his neck and limbs. He had a host of complaints, including severe vomiting and nausea, constipation, frequent episodes of pain in the abdomen, tiredness, and headache. He had been having bouts of intermittent fever for the past six months, but they had recently become worse.

I examined him. Except for the gross weight loss, I could not find any major abnormality. My impression was that Surya had some undiagnosed cancer.

I went through all his papers. His liver and kidney functions were abnormal. His ultrasound scan showed his gallbladder packed with stones [that was what the report said] and was white in appearance. His blood work was normal except for some rise in ESR [Erythrocyte Sedimentation Rate].

The *Mantoux* test [a kind of broad-based test for tuberculosis but by no means diagnostic] was strongly positive. He has had multiple exposures to antibiotics, antacids, and bowel looseners. Presently, the doctors, given his weight loss, episodes of fever, and positive Mantoux test, had advised him to begin a trial of anti-tuberculosis drugs.

This was when he thought of consulting me.

I went through his papers again. There was a marginal increase in his calcium levels in a test done some time back. I ordered a repeat test for blood calcium and parathormone. Both were very high. I also asked my sonologist friend to repeat the ultrasound test. The report came back as milk of calcium in the gallbladder, which had been interpreted as packed gallstones in the previous report.

The diagnosis was obvious now. Surya had a rare condition called parathyroid adenoma. In this condition, the parathyroid glands secrete a hormone called parathormone [PTH] in excess, which causes calcium to move from the bones to blood, and it gets deposited in various tissues and organs, producing a myriad of signs and symptoms.

Further tests, which included a scan of the parathyroid gland using a radioactive substance, proved Surya did have an active tumour of the gland. Removing the tumour under radio-guided local anaesthesia was not difficult for the surgeon.

Parathyroid glands, four of them, are small bean-sized structures located in the periphery and at the back of the thyroid gland. The Thyroid gland is located under the skin in the front of the neck and is partly responsible for the rounded shape of our neck. The thyroid secretes a hormone called thyroxine that acts as a catalyst in the function of each organ in our body. Parathyroid glands produce a hormone called parathormone that controls the calcium and vitamin D metabolism, which are intricately linked.

When the calcium level is high, less parathyroid hormone is produced, and when it is low, more hormone is released into the bloodstream. When both the calcium and parathormone levels are high, one suspects unbridled hyperactivity of the parathyroid gland, as was happening in Surya's case, thus causing many confusing symptoms.

He made an excellent recovery. His vomiting stopped within a week, and he was able to retain food; then his stomach pains stopped, and his bowel movements returned to normal. The liver also returned to normal, and the weakness gradually went. It took three months for the liver to recover and one year for the creatinine levels [kidney function] to return to normal. What about the gallbladder? The opacity was still there when the ultrasound study was repeated a year later, but less intense.

The hyperactivity was due to a non-cancerous tumour of the parathyroid gland, which was promptly diagnosed and effectively treated.

The advantage of a general physician, compared to a specialist, is that he or she looks at the whole body rather than in compartments and thus *occasionally scores*.

❖❖◆❖

The Patient Who Knew Too Much

There are all kinds of patients. We doctors cannot pick and choose. Most of the time they do follow our advice and treatment, but sometimes they don't. Patients have their own reasons and some of them are genuine. Visiting a doctor, however nice he or she may be, can be a stressful experience. There is a term called "white coat hypertension". This means high blood pressure due to seeing a doctor [white coat].

But sometimes the noncompliance can be due to the patient's perception of his or her illness. A person with chronic diseases like diabetes or high blood pressure may feel that going to a doctor is a waste of money and time as he [the doctor] is likely to prescribe the same treatment as before. Sometimes, like I said before, they just want to avoid the stress of seeing the doctor.

Mrs. N doesn't belong to this class and her reason for avoiding coming to see me and thus getting into trouble is too much of misplaced knowledge and self-treatment. Even when one is dealing with chronic illnesses, there is a need to see the doctor periodically as there will be new pharmaceutical and medical developments which will be better than the old ones. Drug treatment of diabetes and high blood pressure has undergone a lot of changes. However, the treatment for low thyroid status remains the same.

Mrs. N is an intelligent woman who successfully runs her own software company. This has made her overconfident and she has this air of *'I know all'* to all problems of life, which includes those related to health.

I had spotted her hypothyroidism when she came to show me her annual medical reports. I had put her on a small dose of thyroid hormone and had asked her to come for dose adjustment after three months, along with the blood reports. She had not turned up. When she did, it was because her husband insisted that she should. This visit was because of loss of weight, tiredness, anxiety and palpitation of some six months duration. I asked her about the thyroid status for which I had initiated treatment some years back.

She said, "That is ok."

I asked her, "When did you do the tests?"

"One year ago," she replied.

"What is the dose you are on?"

"100mcgs daily," she said.

"How did it go from the initial dose of 25 mcgs to 100 mcgs??" I asked her.

"I did the tests every three months and adjusted the dosage. With 100 mcgs the values were normal. So, I have continued the same dose for the past year." she said.

"Did you consult any doctor?" I asked.

She said, "No but I did some research on hypothyroidism and followed the instructions given there. I also take calcium supplements along with it, though you had not recommended them when I met with you last." This she said in an accusing tone. True, one must give calcium supplements concurrently with thyroid hormone medication, which I would have had she come to me for a follow-up.

I did not want to get into an argument with her but now had a clue as to what must have happened since her last visit.

I proceeded to examine her. Her pulse was racing. She was sweating and her hands were trembling. She was also having increased bowel movements—All characteristics of hormone overload, causing overactivity [hyperthyroidism].

Now came the tricky part. How to convince this egocentric woman of the blunder she has committed, without hurting her feelings and her ego? I took the easy way out and told her, "It occasionally happens that what we consider a normal dose can turn out to be an overdose, and this may have happened in your case. I suggest we do the thyroid profile again along with a test for diabetes," and asked her to get back with the reports. Surprisingly, she took it well as I had not directly accused her of harming herself by this over-drugging.

She returned after a week with her reports. Hormone levels were way above normal. She also had altered sugar levels. She was frightened *out of her wits*. I was sure she had done her research and had information overload which had caused and increased her anxiety and distress.

I came straight to the point and told her, "It is easy to control both your sugar and hormone levels but promise me you will follow my advice and not *search Google*. If you have any doubts, ask me in person or on the phone."

She appeared pleased and asked how she had developed diabetes. "I never had it before and no one else in the family has it," she mentioned in an aggrieved tone.

I said, "Too much thyroid hormone sometimes increases the blood sugar. It will settle down and you will not need any medication once the hormone levels are normal."

It took six months for her to get back to normal. Both her hormone and sugar levels returned to normal. Within a year, her weight also returned to normal. Now she need not see me often, but she makes it a point to visit me faithfully once every three months.

❖❖◆❖

Suresh Kumar and his Errant Prostate

When Kumar first visited me around ten years back, it was for his backache. Years of doing a chairbound job with little or no exercise had made his back rigid, and he suffered from chronic lower backache. Like many these days, he did not have a single doctor who took care of all his health problems. He too had drifted to different doctors, which included an orthopaedic and a physiotherapist. He had a sheaf of papers, which included X-rays and MRI scans and various types of medication and physiotherapy exercises.

After going through his papers and examining him, I advised him of some doable lifestyle changes and a daily regimen of spine stretches. He was and is a good patient, and by diligent following, or by his good luck, he got rid of his backache. His confidence in me took a boost, and he began consulting me for all his problems.

He had migrated from Rajasthan and chosen Bangalore to settle with his family. When he first met me, he was in his mid-sixties. After he got cured of his backache, he dropped in one day and told me about another of his problems.

He said, "Doc, of late I am having this gastric trouble."

"What gastric trouble?" I asked.

"I have this burning," he said, pointing to the pit of the stomach. And he continued, "A lot of belching and a vomiting feeling and sometimes a bit of fever."

The symptoms he was having suggested hyperacidity, but hyperacidity does not cause fever.

I asked him, "Have you measured with a thermometer?"

He said "No."

I asked him to do so if he were to get these symptoms again. I prescribed a course of antacids and proton pump inhibitors.

A couple of months later, he was back again. He had all the symptoms as before, and, in addition, had some lower bowel problems like irregular motions.

"What about fever?" I asked.

"Less than 100 degrees but not on all days," he said.

I ordered some tests, including tests for his liver and gallbladder function.

While doing the ultrasound scan of his abdomen, they scanned his prostate [an organ that surrounds the urethra at the bladder base] also. It had a volume of 42 ml, and some urine had stayed back in his bladder despite emptying.

I thought Kumar now had a new problem, in addition to his gastric issue. I told him about the finding of the prostate being enlarged and asked if he had any problems with urination. He said he did have but now it was alright, and he was on medication. This was news to me.

Here is another example of patients not revealing all their problems and giving piecemeal information.

"What medicine and since when?" I asked.

He said, "For two years. I got tested as I had a burning sensation during urination at that time. My PSA [prostate-specific antigen] values were high, but tests showed no cancer; the high PSA was due to infection, and the levels returned to normal after treatment."

He was still on medication and had had four episodes of urinary infection, which he had not told me.

I asked him, "Why did you not see me for this?"

He said he thought it was a matter for a urologist and mentioned a well-known one. As the treatment seemed to be working, I did not argue with him but asked him to see me next time with all his old records.

I thought his gastric symptoms could be due to ulcer disease and got him to do an endoscopic study. He went to Dr. K and got this done. The report said erosive gastritis. No ulcer but some erosions in the lining of the stomach, which explained the symptoms. He was also positive for *Helicobacter Pylori* [an organism causing ulcer disease]. I felt happy that at last, I had the diagnosis to explain his repeated episodes of stomach burning.

I prescribed a ten-day course of anti-*H. pylori* treatment and sent him on his way.

Not even a month had elapsed, he was back again. This time not only did he have symptoms due to his stomach but also burning urination and some discomfort in the area around the base of his penis. This discomfort at the base of the penis made me think if Kumar was having prostatitis [infection of the prostate]. Would this be the reason why he was getting these repeated urinary infections, with the germ sitting in the safe haven of a rather unreachable organ like the prostate?

I was a bit pleased that he had come to see me and had not gone to his friend urologist.

I asked him, "Do you have any fever?"

He said it was, as before, around 100 degrees.

He had been on medications to ease the urine flow since the time he had met with the urologist two years before. I asked him to get a urine test done to find out which antibiotic was a suitable one to prescribe. He had already done that and showed the culture sensitivity report. Except for one, most orally administered antibiotics were of no use.

I discussed the problem and told him about the drug resistance issue. He said, "Doc, I am fed up with taking his medicine; it is not agreeing with me. It is helping me to urinate better, but I have difficulty in getting a proper

70

erection, and my sex life has gone for a six ever since I began this drug."

"Why did you not tell the urologist this?" I asked.

He said he felt embarrassed to tell.

I felt he needed treatment for prostate infection. I started him on an antibiotic and asked him to take it for four weeks as the antibiotic penetration to the prostatic tissue is poor and long-term medication was required.

Two months passed. He was back with his symptoms, both urinary and stomach issues this time. This convinced me that he needed to undergo surgery for easing the urine flow and hopefully to get rid of the infection sitting in the prostate tissue.

I told him the best option was surgery; there may be some side effects, including possible dysfunction of sexual function, but it may result in the cure of this urinary infection and eliminate the need for medication. He said he would consider this option and get back and asked me to speak to his urologist. I called the urologist Dr. D, and we discussed the problem and the feasibility of surgery.

This goes by the name TURP [Trans Urethral Resection of Prostate]. In this procedure, a tunnel is bored through the prostate gland, and the passage for the urine flow is cleared. A successfully done surgery gives long-term relief and would possibly cure his prostate infection.

Dr. D agreed to do the procedure. Kumar underwent TURP without any problem and returned home after four days. The prostate tissue, as is the norm, was sent for histopathological examination.

The result came after a week.

A big surprise awaited us! The biopsy showed a number of granulomata with central caseation [a kind of pus] suggestive of tuberculosis!

71

Now what we should do was the question. When TURP was done, a passage was bored through the prostate gland and much of the tissue was removed, but some was left behind. What if the TB infection was sitting there? We decided to give him a six-month course of anti-TB treatment. He took this treatment well.

It is four years since the surgery and TB treatment; Kumar is now free not only from urinary infections, which he was getting repeatedly before, but also from gastric problems and occasional fever, not to speak of the backache.

A lesson we learnt was that infection in the prostate can cause symptoms of hyperacidity and backache in addition to the urinary symptoms. But the TB sitting in his prostate was the primary cause!

❖❖❖❖

Unmasking the Ulcer Culprit

In 1971, two years into my practice, Narayanaswamy became my patient. He suffered from peptic ulcer disease that had made his life miserable. At that time, we doctors rightly believed that by reducing the effect of gastric acid, we could control the disease.

The method we adopted to diagnose the disease was to make the patient swallow a viscous radio-opaque liquid called barium and take X-rays of its passage down the gullet, stomach, and intestine. If the ulcer was present in these parts, it would show residual dye sticking to the crater, making it visible. This was not a perfect method, but it was all we had in those days.

Doctors of today might laugh at this, as the advent of fibreoptic endoscopes has made the visualisation of the ulcer easy. We also depended on careful history taking, noting when the pain worsened, before or after meals, during the day or night, and whether vomiting occurred. The treatment relied entirely on getting the patient to eat an insipid bland diet, along with large amounts of aluminium hydroxide and sodium bicarbonate.

If the patient was in acute distress, he was admitted and continuously fed an alkali solution through a nasogastric tube with a funnel attached. A nurse would periodically arrive and pour the antacid-laced milk down the funnel into the patient's gullet.

Many of these patients were also used to alcohol, which was considered one of the causes of ulcer disease and so was forbidden.

One such patient was in the hospital when I was the houseman, and he had this contraption of the gastric tube with a funnel attached at one end. I would see a nurse arrive and pour the milk and antacid mix into the funnel. This patient told the nurse not to bother doing this hourly ritual as he was fit enough to reach for the funnel and do the procedure hourly and went on to demonstrate the process. The nurse was only happy to be relieved of this hourly duty.

While on night rounds, I went near the patient to check his pulse and blood pressure and to find out his response to the antacid drip. He was in deep sleep and was not waking up. There was also a strong smell of spirit. I asked the nurse if any spirit was used to clean the skin before giving any injection. She denied using any spirit.

Then the penny dropped. We checked the patient's bedside cupboard and found an empty bottle of *arrack*, a potent locally made brew. The nearly unconscious patient had been pouring the arrack down the tube instead of milk. His inebriation lasted until late next morning.

Many of these patients ended up under the surgeon's scalpel [knife]. The surgery was called partial or complete

73

gastrectomy with gastroduodenal anastomosis. This surgery was common practice for the surgeons of yesteryear, and in my early years, I too am guilty of sending a few of them for this mutilating procedure. In this operation, part or most of the stomach was removed, and the remaining stump was attached to the upper small intestine, the jejunum [a procedure known as gastrojejunostomy].

Our friend Narayanaswamy was now having, in addition to pain, bouts of vomiting that brought out stale undigested food and was also losing weight. This was a sure sign of repeated scarring and obstruction of the duodenum resulting from continuing hyperacidity.

One fine day surgeons decided to operate, and this surgery was performed, removing part of Narayanaswamy's stomach and duodenum. Thus ended Narayanaswamy's ten-year-long struggle with ulcer disease and another, though minor, problem began as a consequence of this rather mutilating surgery which I will come to later.

Around this time, in the 1970s, a new drug appeared. Dr. [later Sir] James Black discovered that while conventional antacids provided relief, it was neither long-lasting nor very effective. His background in physiology and pharmacology led him to believe that blocking the acid-producing cell receptor would provide longer-lasting relief.

He developed cimetidine [Tagamet]. Cimetidine was hailed at the time as a wonder drug, preventing many sufferers from requiring surgery. This drug and its later derivatives provided significant symptomatic relief but did not completely heal ulcers, and long-term use of these H2 receptor blockers was not recommended.

Then, in the 1990s, came drugs called PPIs [Proton Pump Inhibitors] that performed the same function as cimetidine but more effectively. Incidentally, Dr. Black also invented propranolol [the first beta-blocker] used in heart disease and to lower blood pressure. The discovery of these two drugs, cimetidine and propranolol, brought immense riches to the drug company SKF [then Smith Kline & French] but not to Dr. Black, who was an employee of the company. But it did bring him much fame and a well-deserved knighthood.

Now, Dr. Barry James Marshall arrived on the ulcer scene. And the following is his story and that of a germ now called *Helicobacter pylori*:

Barry James Marshall was born September 30, 1951, in Kalgoorlie, a mining town about 400 miles east of Perth, Western Australia. He completed his internship and residency in internal medicine at Queen Elizabeth II Medical Centre [Sir Charles Gairdner Hospital] in Perth. In 1981, he met J. Robin Warren, a pathologist. Marshall, seeking a research topic, learnt that Warren had a list of patients whose gastric biopsies showed "curved" bacteria. Warren needed a clinician to follow these patients to determine their diagnoses and subsequent progress.

In their meeting, Warren showed slides of the curved bacteria and the histological features of the gastric mucosa. Marshall was aware of the finding of *Campylobacter jejuni* [now renamed *Helicobacter*] as a cause of food-borne gastroenteritis. He noted that the *Campylobacter* organisms appeared very similar to the curved bacilli that Warren had reported in his gastric biopsies.

In early 1983, he contacted Dr. Martin Skirrow, a gastroenterologist at the Worcester Infirmary in England, who subsequently invited him to present his work at the European *Campylobacter* Meeting in Brussels. Marshall visited Skirrow in England, where he saw that peptic ulcer patients there, too, had the spiral organism in their biopsies, just as he had seen in Australia.

Marshall was unsuccessful in developing an animal model, so he decided to experiment on himself. In 1984, following a baseline endoscopy that showed a normal gastric mucosa, he drank a culture of the organism. Three days later, he developed nausea and achlorhydria. Vomiting occurred, and on day 8, a repeat endoscopy and biopsy showed marked gastritis and a positive *H. pylori* culture. On day 14, a third endoscopy was performed, and he then began treatment with antibiotics and bismuth. He recovered promptly and thus fulfilled *Koch's postulates,* proving the role of *H. pylori* in gastritis.

In 1994, the National Institutes of Health held a consensus meeting in Washington, D.C., that concluded with a statement to the effect that the key to the treatment of gastric and duodenal ulcers was the detection and eradication of *H. pylori*. He shared the Nobel Prize in Physiology or Medicine in 2005 with J. Robin Warren.

In the last two decades, advancements in effective *Helicobacter pylori* therapy have revolutionised ulcer disease outcomes, making gastrojejunostomy a rarity. As one general surgeon remarked at one of the professional meetings, Barry Marshall took away the bread and butter from surgeons!

It took an inquisitive young doctor, his dogged perseverance, and ultimately experimenting on himself to convince the sceptical medical community that *Helicobacter pylori* is indeed the cause of peptic ulcer disease, in the *true Hunterian tradition*.

Now let us see what happened to Narayanaswamy post-surgery. Five years after the surgery, he came to see me with weakness and tiredness. He had lost some weight and was found to be anaemic. Tests revealed a blood picture suggestive of both iron and B12 deficiency.

Stomach acid and a hormone called intrinsic factor are produced by the lining of the stomach. In many patients who undergo this surgery, the part of the stomach that secretes these two essential substances is removed, and these patients develop iron and/or B12 deficiency.

Narayanaswamy had a deficiency of both. He recovered with iron and B12 supplements. He is in his seventies and comes twice a year for his B12 injections. But his stomach remains truncated, and he needs to eat small meals!

✥✥✦✥✥

Two Patients, Two Different Outcomes

Angina is a word derived from Latin, related to the words *angere* [to strangle] and *pectus* [chest]. The term describes a sensation of 'strangling' or 'choking' in the chest.

The heart is an extraordinary organ. This bundle of muscle and nerve starts beating a few weeks after conception and continues to beat until death, whether that occurs a hundred years later or sooner, as in the case of a massive heart attack! Its rhythmic beats pump blood to all parts of the body, including some for its own needs.

To meet the heart's demands, there are three main blood vessels. These are named according to their position on the surface of the heart: anterior descending, circumflex, and posterior descending. The first two originate from a common starting point called the main trunk.

As the arteries age and sometimes due to other factors, the *lumen* [space inside heart vessels] becomes gradually narrow, and the blood supply gets compromised. This produces various symptoms which go by the name angina, and the process is called ischaemic heart disease [IHD].

Though the Latin description of a choking chest is appropriate for some forms of angina, there are other presentations, which can include radiating pain down the arm or feeling breathless on exertion, such as climbing stairs. The high degree of clinical suspicion, combined with the easy availability of tests, makes the diagnosis of IHD easy.

Unlike in yesteryear, when advances in imaging technology and interventions [both surgical and medical] were not available, nowadays it is relatively easy to diagnose, and in most cases, to treat. The challenge clinicians face is motivating and convincing patients of the seriousness of the disease, especially when the presenting symptoms are vague. This also depends on the trust patients have in their referring and treating doctors.

I will illustrate this with two examples. In one, the patient implicitly believed what I said and underwent the procedure; in the other, the patient, who was not convinced, went shopping for opinions and ultimately experienced significant morbidity and a compromised quality of life.

The first case is Mr. Sunil Mirchandani. Sunil was in his late forties when he became my patient. Sunil is a British Indian who had business interests in India and had made Bangalore his city of residence. He travelled extensively and led an active social life.

One day, on his way to his office, he came to see me.

I asked him, "What is the problem?"

"No problem, but I've been having these burps with some discomfort in the pit of my stomach," he said.

"Since when?" I asked him.

"Since a few weeks, and it is more after my meals," he replied.

"Have you tried any medication?" I asked.

"Yes, I have tried Gelusil [a popular antacid]."

"Did you get any relief?"

"Not much, Doc," was the response.

I made him lie down and examined him. His blood pressure was normal, and I could not find any abnormality.

I wanted to exclude gallbladder-related illness, which can produce after-dinner symptoms like in Sunil's case. I asked him to get an ultrasound scan done along with a few other tests, and as an afterthought added an ECG [Electrocardiogram].

He returned two days later. All the tests were normal except the ECG. It was abnormal. With the resting ECG itself being abnormal, I felt it risky to subject him to further tests like exercise testing [TMT, Treadmill Test] to confirm a diagnosis and plan the treatment.

I explained the situation to Sunil and told him he needed an angiogram to determine the appropriate treatment, which might include CABG surgery [Coronary Artery Bypass Grafting].

He asked, "Doc, how urgent is it? Can I travel back to London? I have a close friend who is a cardiologist."

I told him the sooner the better. He took the next flight back.

He came to see me two months later and looked as fit as ever.

I asked him, "How are you?"

"Can't be better Doc, I got the surgery done." He showed a lengthy scar extending from his neck to the pit of the stomach and another one on his leg from where they had harvested a vein. He was on some medication. His post-meal symptoms had gone, and except for some tightness due to the healing scar, he was in good shape. I told him so.

He asked me, "Doc, I have come to ask you if I can resume tennis." I told him to do it gradually. Initially slow doubles and after a few weeks, singles.

I also asked him to do an exercise TMT.

He said, "I have already done so," and showed the test records. He was able to exercise the full ten minutes.

I told him to go ahead with his tennis, both singles and doubles, whole hog.

He lived here for a few more years and then returned to London. I lost touch with him, but I wouldn't be surprised if he is still alive and in good health.

Now coming to the second patient, Mr. Ananthram. Ananthram was a business executive and like Sunil M, led a busy life, both professional and social. His wife hailed from Karnataka, and he from Hyderabad, and the couple had lot of relatives, both here and in Hyderabad.

Ananthram suffered from seasonal asthma, which was well-controlled with a combination of inhaled steroids and bronchodilators. He required this treatment for a few months each year. Lately, he had become somewhat of an expert in using [misusing?] these inhalers and rarely consulted me for his asthma. Therefore, when he came to see me after a lapse of nearly a year, it was a bit of a surprise.

I asked him what made him come.

He said, "Doc, this asthma is not getting under control."

But he was not in any distress and was breathing normally. I told him so.

He said, "No Doc, the attacks come once in a way and that too when I climb stairs. I have tried increasing the inhaler dosage but that is not helping."

This man was self-medicating, thinking his breathlessness was due to asthma.

Ananthram has a strong family history of IHD. He had lost his father due to a heart attack. I examined him. Though his blood pressure and heart were normal, and his lungs were clear, I was convinced that Ananthram's problem was angina presenting as breathlessness. I told him the need for an urgent cardiology consult and gave him a letter to a cardiologist friend of mine.

Either Ananthram did not appreciate the seriousness of the situation, did not believe me, or I failed to convince him. He wasted a couple of months, and when he went to Hyderabad on an errand, he consulted a physician friend of his. Instead of making an urgent referral, that doctor wasted more valuable time ordering further tests, including a TMT.

During the TMT, Ananthram became breathless and complained of severe chest pain. The TMT was aborted, and he was admitted to the hospital. The TMT showed that he already had suffered a heart attack, which fortunately had not caused extensive damage and had gone unnoticed.

Had he had one when he came to see me? One never knows.

He then suffered a second, more serious heart attack. Though he recovered, his quality of life suffered, and he had to be treated for chronic heart failure. He was on multiple medications and constant supervision till his death some ten years later.

Had he followed my advice and sought treatment, he would have avoided the subsequent heart attack and possibly not have developed the heart failure that ultimately led to his premature death.

❖❖❖❖

Life, Loss, Laughter and a Lot of Four-Letter Words
It was more than twenty years since I had last seen Luke [Lukas], and naturally, I was pleased when he came. Many times, I am unaware of the reason why my patients stay away from me for such long periods, especially people like Luke, who need to see a doctor periodically to check their blood pressure. It has been my practice not to ask why they have not seen me, as long as they are getting adequate attention.

81

What disturbs me, however, is when this is not the case, and they simply quit or continue taking the medications prescribed when they last saw me. This often has unpleasant, and sometimes disastrous, consequences.

Luke must have been pushing sixty when this incident occurred. During his younger days, he was a university-level athlete and a good hockey player. After spending several years abroad, he returned to India and settled in Bangalore. He would periodically visit Mangalore to spend time with his elderly parents. I had even, on occasion, seen them when they visited him here.

Luke enjoyed life, and whenever he came, he somehow managed to make me laugh. His conversation was peppered with the frequent use of four-letter swear words, and he used them liberally to make his point, even when he came to get himself examined.

So, naturally, I was happy to see him return and asked him how he had been.

He said, "Doc, I am now in Mangalore, in my ancestral home. I sold my house here and moved there. I am sorry I couldn't meet you before I left."

I refrained from asking him how his wife and two sons were doing. The sons must be well into their late twenties by now. I, as a matter of policy, do not make this natural enquiry because I don't know what can of worms I might open by doing so. Often, during the intervening period, unpleasant things would have happened, and the person would not want to be reminded of them. If the happenings are pleasant, they will tell me of their own accord. So, I kept quiet.

But this doesn't prevent my patients from asking me. Luke too was no exception and asked, "How is your family doing?"

I narrated all that had happened to my family in the intervening period. He said, "Doc, you look bloody good."

I said, "Thanks."

"Are not you going to ask about my f........g family?" he asked.

I kept quiet. "So, you know about them," Luke said.

I told him I had no clue as to what had happened to him and his family since I last met him, which was more than twenty years. He then proceeded to tell me the sad story of the misfortune he suffered mainly due to his f......g sons and his bl.......y wife supporting them. In short, they had done badly in life and were an economic burden on him in his old age. I did not want to know the details.

I asked him why he had come to see me. He said, "You know me very well. I cannot sleep, I am always worried and my doctor there gives me sleeping pills which do me no bl...y good, and all the time I am thinking of my two f......g sons who have become experts in converting food into shit. You want to know something more? They have, between them, b....red me so hard and for so long that I can't even fart without pain."

Typical of Luke, even in his misery he makes others laugh.

He had depression, which I was able to treat, and now he is managing well despite the continuing problems.

❖❖◆❖

Red Herring
(Written some years back)

Often, we doctors go astray chasing the wrong diagnosis and causing avoidable distress to our patients. This is one such story which happened in my practice.

I am now treating the fourth generation of Pillays. The old man Pillay, who came to Bangalore from the state of Kerala some sixty years back, died many years ago. The young man in question is a twenty-five-year-old grandson who is employed as an engineer in a private company.

He suffers from kidney stone disease and periodically develops pain in his back, along the ureter's path [the tube that drains urine from the kidney to the bladder], down his flank to his groin, and ends up either with me or at the nearby hospital's outpatient department.

He developed one such episode of severe backache and ended up in the hospital. A scan of his abdomen revealed kidney stones, though *none* was visible in the ureters. Based on the history, he was given painkillers and asked to come the next day. He did not get better and developed urinary urgency and frequency, and constipation. The physician thought the urinary symptoms to be due to possible infection and suggested a urine study. The patient's complaint of constipation was attributed to taking painkillers, and his feeling of tingling sensations in his legs to anxiety. Pending urine study, he was given antibiotics and sent home.

He came over to see me the next day. His back pain was localised and on both sides. He had abnormal pain and touch sensations and there was improper control of his bladder. Also, he was unable to evacuate his bowels. Examination revealed grossly abnormal neurological signs in both lower legs, and there was bladder and bowel involvement. I was dealing with a serious illness called *Transverse Myelitis* which needed urgent expert management.

Myelitis is a general term used to describe all inflammatory conditions that affect the sheath [cover] of the nerves and nerve cells. It can be due to infection or immunological insult. The latter was the case with this young man, and he was saved from the dire consequences of possible paralysis of his body from navel downwards by massive doses of steroids and only a week's hospitalisation.

He made a very good recovery.

He still has stones in the substance of the kidney, but these are sitting quietly for the present.

❖❖◆❖

ICU: I Care for You

It was on the 28th of August 2014 that this incident took place. My close friend and neighbour, Nanjappa dropped in to show me his blood reports and chest X-ray. As it was in the afternoon, he came to the main door of the house. There were two friends of mine sitting in the drawing room. Nanjappa knew these two persons. On seeing them, instead of acknowledging or greeting them, he gave a vacant, stupid-looking smile. One of the friends asked him, "How are you?" He replied, looking at me instead of the friend who spoke, "Doctor."

I knew then that something was amiss; this was not normal behaviour. I took him to my examination room and asked, "You know who those two are?" He again gave me a vacant smile and was obviously at a loss.

Nanjappa suffered from periodic mild episodes of bronchospasm and responded well to the inhaled combination of bronchodilators and steroids. He had come two days before and there was a slight fever in addition to the wheeze. I was thinking of starting an antibiotic, but before that to make sure it was not a bacterial infection, I had asked for the tests, the reports of which he had now come to show. He looked unwell, and a quick check of his lungs showed widespread sounds, and he continued to have a fever. This plus his odd behaviour led me to diagnose delirium due to lung infection despite normal X-ray and blood picture.

This was indeed an emergency, and I rushed him to the hospital after getting in touch with Dr. R, who was the head of one of the medical units. Dr. R assured me that the resident at the emergency would take care of the patient. In the emergency department, the work was fast and furious. The bedside PO2 showed a level of 56, and the ECG was bizarre. This, with the rattling chest in a seventy-plus-year-old, the first thought was that he was in acute heart failure, and my telling the young resident that he had this LBBB [Left Bundle Branch Block] ECG pattern for many years did not convince him [and I don't blame him one bit].

He went ahead and ordered the necessary tests, the results of which showed sodium levels of 120 [very low] and normal cardiac enzymes.

Now the doctors were convinced that this was not a heart attack but an acute lung infection with spasm and respiratory distress with electrolyte disturbance. Appropriate measures were instituted and naturally, he was admitted to the ICU [Intensive Care Unit].

Now another drama began. I got a call from Nanjappa at 10 pm that night. He said, "Doc, am I going to die?"

I asked him why he thought so.

He said, "They have put me in the ICU, and the patient in the next bed died just now."

"Didn't the doctor tell you what your problem is?" I asked.

He said, "One young doctor told me that I have a lung infection and *electrolysis*."

He meant electrolyte abnormality.

It took me fifteen minutes to explain what the problem was and why he was not going to die. His last request was for me to use my influence and get him out of the deathly ICU. After taking this promise from me, thankfully, he hung up.

The next day, my friend Dr. R could only talk to me late afternoon when he could find some time. I told him about my friend's request.

He said, "Your friend, though better now, is not responding to inhaled steroids given through a nebuliser. I have started him on intravenous antibiotics, and he needs to be in the intensive care for a few more days. I will shift him to the semi-ICU as soon as possible where he will be more comfortable."

I thought I saw the end of my friend's problem. But I was mistaken. A call came from my friend two days later. One problem with mobile phones is their easy accessibility.

He said, "Doc, they are keeping me here in this different ICU and have not shifted me to the ward. Here too there are very sick patients. Next to me is one of them; he coughs non-stop. I am afraid I will end up getting another and more serious disease if I continue to be here."

His concerns were genuine, and I told him I would investigate this.

The problem we family doctors face when a patient of ours gets admitted to hospital is communicating and following up with the consultant concerned. Many hospitals have this ladder of hierarchy, and while the junior doctors bear the brunt of routine work, they generally cannot give accurate information, and even if they do, they cannot often take decisions like this one – shifting from semi-ICU to the ward.

Again, I waited for my friend Dr. R to return my call. I had to wait till late evening to get his call. I told him the problem.

He updated me like this: "I had to begin oral steroids, and Mr. Nanjappa's diabetes has gotten out of control, and now I am struggling with his infection, asthma, and diabetes. You please advise him to put up with the discomfort for two more days, and I will shift him to a room."

I called my friend next morning and asked him, "How are you?"

He said, "They want me to be in this place for two more days. They have put a mobile screen around my bed now. I hope *this will protect me from getting infected.*"

I couldn't help but laugh. Usually, such screens are put around the bed of a very seriously ill patient so that the other occupants need not witness the gory scenes that sometimes occur in these ICU wards. In my friend's case, it was the reverse, so that he need not see the other's serious condition – that much credit for my influence.

He duly recovered and came home.

He had three similar episodes, but fortunately, not as serious as the first one, all the same – needing oral steroids, antibiotics, worsening of diabetes, and use of insulin. I was able to take him off the insulin, taper his prednisolone to 5 mg a day, and put him back on the old dose of metformin.

A pulmonology consultation was of no help. Looking for any pre-existing cause also showed no results. His IgE [Immunoglobulin E] levels were normal, and his lung function was near normal. Why he got these in this characteristic pattern remained an enigma.

And whenever he fell ill, I felt it would have been better that I had fallen ill instead because of the tensions I had to go through!

Taking unbiased care of close friends and relatives is always difficult. The worst thing is that they don't know this and will not allow us to get someone else to take care of them.

Mr. Nanjappa is no more. In his death I lost a close friend.

✦✦✦✦

2

DIAGNOSED AT FIRST SIGHT

Simple 'Solution'

Mr. Sudheendra is a seventy-year-old retired engineer who is mildly diabetic, hypertensive, and on medication. He underwent a successful coronary artery bypass surgery eight years back and since then he has been seeing me twice a year without fail.

Lately, however, he has not been able to keep up with this schedule for various reasons. One of them is the strong rumour that I have given up practice and have gone away to the United States to be with my daughter. To substantiate this, Sudheendra had on several occasions found my consulting chambers locked, with my neighbours informing him that I had stopped the practice.

While the first rumour has no basis, the second has some truth to it. Two years ago, I made a deliberate decision to be available only to those who book prior appointments and to keep the doors open only at those times and closed at all other times. This information, given to my well-meaning neighbours, resulted in their informing those who came without an appointment and found the doors shut, that I had quit practice!

Be that as it may, let me get back to Mr. Sudheendra. He joyfully, [according to him] found out that I am alive and kicking and have not stopped seeing patients. And thus, there he was in front of me.

After the usual pleasantries, I asked him, "What is the problem?"

"I am extremely tired, can't even walk half a kilometre," he said.

"Since when?" I asked.

"In the past two weeks," he replied.

"What have you been doing in the last two weeks?" I asked.

"Fearing the worst, I went to see my cardiologist and got tests done."

He showed me the cardiology test reports and the prescription. All the reports were normal, and he was told not to worry, to take the vitamin pills, and to get back when due.

I proceeded to examine him. Like his cardiologist, I too found his pulse and blood pressure normal, with no evidence of heart failure. Now I am faced with the problem of why Sudheendra is having this recent onset of tiredness.

A thought occurred. Could he be having low sodium levels? He gave no history of vomiting, diarrhoea, or recent infection which could have caused his low sodium level and weakness.

"How much water are you drinking?" I asked.

"At least two litres in the morning and maybe another two during the day," he replied.

"No doctor, more than that. As it is now summer, he is always drinking," chimed in his wife.

"Are you on a low-salt diet?" was my next question.

"Yes doctor, since my surgery I have been on a low-salt diet."

Here is a possible explanation for Mr. S's tiredness. The onset of summer, high fluid intake, and a low-salt diet resulting in *hyponatremia* [low sodium] might have caused the tiredness.

I asked him to get his blood electrolytes checked urgently, to drink a glass of lime juice with half a teaspoon of salt three times a day, and to restrict his water intake while we waited for the results.

"But then doctor, his blood pressure will go up if he takes so much of salt." This was the wife's worry.

"Unlikely in the short run," I reassured her.

With that, they took their leave.

Three days passed, and there was no news from Sudheendra or his wife. This worried me. Had I missed anything? Was the patient alright or in serious trouble? Was he in hospital? These were unpleasant thoughts.

I called him. His wife took the call, and I asked her, "How is your husband doing?"

"*Daaktre* [doctor in Kannada], he is perfectly normal and has now gone for his walk. I wanted to ask you how long he needs to take this extra salt?" she replied.

"What about the test results?" I asked.

"We did not go, as he was feeling normal," she said and wanted to know if he still needed to do the tests.

Two weeks of illness got cured by *two teaspoons of salt!*

❖❖◆❖

From Vanity to Vexation

This young woman, Poornima has been coming to me since her school days. Now, married, she has settled in Mumbai and visits Bangalore once or twice a year to see her parents and siblings. Since her marriage a couple of years ago and her moving away, her visits have become rare, though she calls me once in a while to get some advice related to her health.

This time, however, it was for a problem that had been bugging her for some time. She started having an itchy rash on her right eyelid six months back. Initially, it was mild but as the days went by it became more severe and there was some discharge over the rash. Lately, it had appeared over her left eyebrow.

"How long has it been there?" I asked Poornima.

"Six months, Doctor, and it is becoming worse lately and has spread to my left eyelid also," she said.

"Did not you seek help from your doctor?" I asked.

"I did, first with my family doctor, and he prescribed some ointment. It helped a bit, but he later sent me to a skin specialist. He prescribed a different one to be applied in the morning and another one in the evening."

While we were talking, I noticed, Poornima constantly touching her eyebrows and nose with her hands and fingers. On a closer look, I felt there was some redness and thickening on the tip of her nose, and the right eyelid was covered with a scaly rash which had thickened the skin. A thinner version was on her left eyelid.

I asked her, "Since when are you wearing this nail paint?"

"Many years doctor," she said.

"Have you changed it recently?" I asked.

"I keep changing the nail paint constantly, Doctor" was her answer.

I began to wonder if the nail polish was the cause of her continuing skin allergy. Was she carrying the allergen from her nail to the eyelid and nose?

I asked her, "Can you stop using the nail paint?"

"I will do anything to get rid of this hideous rash," she said.

With this promise, she went away.

I got a call from her a fortnight later, profusely thanking me. Her rashes had almost gone, and she wanted to know if she could restart using her nail paint!

I asked her if she wanted the rash *back*.

There was an emphatic no. Her nail painting days were over and so was her eyelid rash.

❖❖❖❖

A Colourful Diagnosis

I got a call. "This is Kamini calling from Delhi".

"Which Kamini?" I asked, as there are three whom I know.

"Kamini Mehrotra," she said.

This Kamini is a thirty-year-old mother of two children and an occasional patient of mine.

"What is the problem?" I asked.

"I'm having it again," she said.

"What is it that you're having again?"

"The same old urinary infection. This time I'm also passing blood," she said.

I told her to see a doctor urgently.

"I have, Doctor. He wants to admit me."

I told her that she just needed a urine check and maybe a scan, and that admission might not be required.

"Doc, I'm taking the evening flight back and will see you tomorrow morning."

She didn't turn up. I thought she must have seen some other doctor and got herself treated. Matters rested there for a month.

She called once again and said, "I'm passing *bloody* urine again."

"Any pain, fever, frequency?" I asked.

She said, "None of these, but only red urine."

I asked her, "Last time, did you get any tests done?"

"No," she said. "It wasn't blood in the urine, but my period mixed with urine. I went to my gynaecologist, and by then it had stopped."

"Get a urine sample tested," I said.

As the examination was normal, and this wasn't her menstruation time, I wanted to exclude serious kidney disease.

She called in the evening. "Doc, I've sent the report by WhatsApp. Just have a look and call me."

The report showed no red cells [blood], but the colour was pink. There was no evidence of infection. No blood, but the colour was pink. Otherwise, normal.

The penny dropped. I called her. "Did you eat beetroot salad last night?"

"No, Doctor, but I ate *dragon fruit*. Come to think of it, I ate dragon fruit last time also when this happened."

That was likely the answer, so I looked up the literature and found that dragon fruit can, of course, cause red-coloured urine.

I called Kamini and told her what I had found; there was no need for any urine culture test or a scan.

Another lesson learnt.

❖❖◆❖

Arunima Ghosh and her Ringworm

Arunima and her husband Aloke, like many Bengalis, have made Bangalore their home. Like many outsiders, they too are successful and Arunima can be called an upper-class socialite. She was in her early thirties when she became my patient. She had inherited high blood pressure from her parents and needed to see me periodically. She was good-looking and always dressed in the latest fashion, even when it meant visiting the doctor's clinic.

I was a bit surprised to see her, as her regular appointment wasn't due. I asked her what had happened.

She said, "Doctor, I have developed this ringworm patch," and showed me a red ring-shaped rash on the inner side of her upper arm. As she wore a sleeveless blouse, it indeed looked ugly, and I could understand her worry on two counts. One was this ringworm [a kind of common fungal infection of the skin], and the other was its location, which made her wearing a sleeveless blouse impossible.

I asked her, "How long have you had this?"

She said, "Nearly three months. Now it has become bigger."

"Does it itch?" I asked. She said no.

To me, it did not look like ringworm. I told her so and asked her, "How come you think it is ringworm?"

She said, "My friend told me. She too had a similar rash and got cured by applying ringworm ointment."

Curious, I asked her, "Have you applied it too?"

She replied, "Yes, but it has not helped."

If she had left it alone and come, it would have been easier to diagnose. But she had applied this antifungal ointment, which had some small amount of steroid, and the nature of the rash was tough to diagnose. I told a slightly embarrassed Arunima not to apply any ointment for a week and come back.

She came back after ten days, this time she wore a blouse with a sleeve, which meant that the culprit was still very much there on the skin of her upper arm.

Now it was quite clear. This patch of skin ailment was psoriasis. For the next fifteen minutes, I told her about psoriasis and the many problems it can cause, including the involvement of joints and the like. After listening to me, she said, "It is only a small rash; you prescribe some ointment to hide this so that I can wear my proper dress." By this, she meant a sleeveless blouse.

I felt all my lecture was a waste. This woman was only interested in her wearing a sleeveless blouse and obviously thought, I was making a big issue of a small patch.

I did not see her for six months.

Then one day she came with complaints of vomiting and loose bowels. Mild infection following her eating out. Easy enough to treat, I asked her, "What has happened to your rash?" She showed the area where the patch was. It was barely visible.

I asked her, "Are you applying the ointment that I had prescribed?"

She said no, but was applying *bhasma* [a kind of ash] given to her by ….*Baba* [a holy man] and it had worked wonders.

I have often come across this kind of patients. They take delight in telling me how an alternative system [naturopathy, homeopathy, *anypathy*] that they had followed, worked, indirectly telling me that mine did not. Mostly, these are for come-and-go illnesses, but occasionally, and for me inexplicably, a genuine cure has come about where I have not succeeded.

Arunima's psoriasis was one such illness. It has these waxing and waning periods. It may completely disappear, only to appear again. I refrained from telling her this, as she would not have believed me in any case. I complimented her and her ability now to wear her favourite dresses. She went beaming.

Some more months passed.

Arunima arrived, and I could see she was very worried. I asked her. Showing her arm, she said, "This *bhooth* [ghost] has come back. Now I have another one near my lower leg and a small one behind my ear."

I repeated my earlier explanation and told her to continue using the two ointments [one containing salicylic acid and another containing a steroid] and to await remission.

This time, she accepted my advice, and as her psoriatic lesions were localised, she did not come to any great harm over the years when she was my patient.

I must tell readers that this episode was before the advent of Methotrexate and TNF [Tumour Necrosis Factor] inhibitors.

❖❖❖❖

A Lump of Worry

New patients are naturally wary of the doctor and vice versa. They do not know what they are going to get with the consult. It may not be a pleasant experience for either party. Who knows, in a worst-case scenario, the doctor may not hesitate to pass a death sentence on the hapless patient.

This patient, who gate-crashed [came without a prior appointment] into my clinic, had severe anxiety writ large on his face. I asked him to sit and try to relax. He sat on the front of the chair, and I could see his hands trembling. He was also perspiring.

I waited for him to begin. After a minute or so he said, "I have a *tumour* on the lower part of my back, and it is hurting me."

Normally patients don't say tumour; they say swelling or lump. If someone says tumour, I am certain he has already seen another doctor and has borrowed the terminology.

We doctors, as a tribe, don't know [or don't want to] how to put our diagnosis in simple lingo. We have to say Myocardial Infarction instead of heart attack, and Cholecystitis instead of infected gallbladder. Sometimes when we don't know how to describe an illness appropriately enough with a high-sounding name, like when one has dizzy spells due to vestibular disease, then we call it BPPV which stands for benign paroxysmal positional vertigo, which in real terms means a benign form of vertigo that comes in paroxysms related to the position of the head!

So, this "tumour" word had me worried because it connotes a growth of some type and could be serious especially when it is also causing backache. After getting the history that the swelling had been noticed several years ago and the pain had been present for the past two months, I asked him to undress and lie down on the couch.

This is what I found. He had a small, mobile lump, and he had a stiff lower back. The lump belonged to a group of fibro-fatty, benign tumours called fibromas/lipomas. The rigid back needed to be investigated. I told him so and assured him that the two were unrelated. He said he had done a lot of tests, which included an MRI [magnetic resonance imaging] scan. He proceeded to take out a sheaf of papers from his sling bag. The MRI showed a slightly indented cord but not serious enough to have caused his backache. His other reports were normal.

What this young man needed was posture correction at work and a set of exercises to stretch his lower back. His lump needed no intervention. I told him so.

"Doctor, are you *sure*?" he asked.

"As sure as one can be, based on the evidence," I said. Then he took out another set of papers in which a surgeon had advised admission for removal of the tumour and surgery for the disc prolapse!

I sat in silence for a while, not knowing what to do or say. I told him, "You have come to me for an opinion and advice, and according to me you need no surgery. Try out these exercises, get back to me after six weeks, and we will review your back problem. The lipoma [lump] needs no removal—not now and not in the foreseeable future."

That was some time prior. He came to see me again. His backache was much better, and his much-feared lump did not seem to bother him.

❖❖◆❖

A Prescription for Peace

When I first saw Ramamoorthy, he was a school-going youngster. Except for the usual minor illness episodes, he was in good health. When he was in college, the family moved to a different part of the city, and I introduced them to a friend of mine, Dr. S, who practised in that area. I had heard that he had done well in life and was the HR chief of a multinational company.

So, it was a surprise to get a call from his wife Suchithra, requesting an appointment. She also warned me that it would take some time. To my question about their going to my friend Dr. S, she said she would tell me about it later.

The party arrived on the agreed date and time. I say party because, along with Ramamoorthy and his wife, his mother-in-law and father-in-law had come along too. Normally one does not see so many attendants, especially in-laws. When asked, they said they had some work in the neighbourhood and therefore they had come along. This was an obvious lie, as the real reason was some anxiety associated with the son-in-law's health and to support the very anxious daughter.

I made them wait outside and called the couple in. I had not seen Ramamoorthy since his wedding. Except for some weight gain, he looked quite normal to my eyes.

I asked him, "What is the matter with you? You look all right to me."

Before he could open his mouth, Suchithra intervened, "Doctor, he will not say anything, but I know something is wrong with him."

"What is wrong?" I asked her.

"Since the last six months, his headache has become worse. He has become quiet, and he hardly sleeps. I took him to your friend. He only asked us to diet and exercise and get an opinion from Dr. K, his friend, a psychiatrist. We went there and that doctor gave him some medicine that this man refuses to take properly. I am at a loss to know what to do." A torrent of words in one breath.

Now it was Ramamoorthy's turn. I asked him.

He said, "I am OK, Doctor."

Before he could proceed further, Suchithra intervened and said, "Doctor, I will wait outside. If I am here, he may not tell you his problem." Saying so, she thankfully left the scene.

He began, "Doctor, I am well, but it is difficult to convince her. She means well but is convinced that I am unwell. This is

100

because of my occasional headache and my giving this as an excuse to retire to my room."

I asked him, "Why did you do that?"

"Doctor, you don't know Suchithra. As soon as I get back from the office, she will start her talk, and this goes on and on. I need to be alone for some time and I need to work from home often, though it is not always. The only time she leaves me alone is when I complain of a headache. Then I can carry on with my work uninterrupted."

"But then this is her other complaint that you work too much despite having this headache. Have you told this to Dr. S?" I asked.

"Yes, I did, but he believes in Suchithra and not in me. Both have even got my CT brain scan done and as expected, it was clear," he replied.

"So, you don't get headaches at all?" I asked.

"No Doctor, I do get them now once in a way. I consulted with you when I was in college, and you had given me simple paracetamol. It is not that frequent or serious to worry about. I made the mistake of taking this as an excuse to get some time for myself at home. Now no one believes me. Suchithra is so anxious about my health that she seems to be panicking over small problems. For a month or so, her parents have joined in this *chorus* too."

I wanted to hear from my friend Dr. S. So, I took the phone and called him.

He said, "Don't let him fool you. He has depression and anxiety. Dr. K also thinks so. He has a responsible job, and we feel he finds it difficult to handle the work pressure. The problem is that he refuses to take medication as he thinks it is harmful. His wife is trying her best."

So, my friend too was convinced. Now where do I stand? I thought for a while and decided to talk to Suchithra. I called her inside and asked Ramamoorthy to wait outside.

I told her, "Your husband seems to carry some problem or the other in his head when he comes home. Therefore, he becomes absent-minded and quiet when he is sorting out these problems. If he is disturbed at that time, his headaches may become worse and interfere with his sleep. What I suggest is, when he comes home, give him a cup of coffee and for the next hour or two, leave him alone to his ways. Let us do this experiment for the next two weeks."

"We will review after two weeks; let him not take any medicines in these two weeks," I added.

I assured her that nothing serious would happen if he did not take the drugs for the next two weeks. She agreed reluctantly, as the psychiatrist had warned her why it was important for the patient to take the medication, as depression is a very serious illness and can lead to suicide, *etc.*

Thus, the laborious interview ended after an hour.

Two weeks went by. The party did not turn up. Both Suchithra and Ramamoorthy called and thanked me separately. Things were much better in their household.

❖❖◆❖

Dermatitis Medicamentosa

I have known Shabbar since his school days. His father Salim retired from government service and settled in my practice area. It was a well-educated family. Shabbar too, like his father, grew to be a well-mannered young man but unlike his father, he took to business and within a couple of years, became quite wealthy going by the standards prevailing thirty years ago. His wife Ayesha too came from an educated family, and it was a pleasure to see this couple.

102

Shabbar's business needed him to travel out of the city and in one of his travels this happened. In his own words it was an accident. *Achanak* is the Urdu word he used. This *achanak* meant that he engaged in unprotected sex with a sex worker when he was away on one of his business trips.

When he came to see me, it was nearly six months after the episode. I knew something serious was worrying him. Normally a happy-go-lucky youngster, he was restless and sweating.

I asked him, "What is the problem?"

"Doctor *Saab*, I do not know where to begin, I have an STD."

STD is the short form for sexually transmitted diseases. Normally, this abbreviation is used by doctors, so I wondered why this fellow was using it.

I asked him. He took out a sheaf of papers and placed them in front of me. These were case notes and prescriptions from three doctors, including a skin and venereal disease specialist. There were also blood test reports. All the reports were negative for STDs. Several courses of antibiotics and many ointments for local use have been tried but had not given him relief.

I told him, "You have no venereal disease [STD]."

"But then, why am I having this problem?" he asked.

"What problem?"

"I have pain, that [meaning his penis] had become red, and when I have sex, I have severe pain and it is having an effect on my wife, and she is screaming at me." He used a slang word [*voh bambdi maarthi*].

I asked him to undress and then I examined him. There was redness over the glans and a bit on the skin. After cleaning with soap and removing the ointment he had applied, the redness became even more obvious.

In the past, we called this condition "Dermatitis Medicamentosa" [a rash caused by medication].

I advised him to stop all medications oral and local, to wash with ordinary soap and water, to refrain from sexual activity for two weeks, and if he did not improve, to come and see me.

Within two weeks, he became normal, and happiness once again prevailed with Shabbar and Ayesha.

❖❖◆❖

Belliappa's Backache

Many years ago, I was the zonal medical officer for Hindustan Aeronautics Limited [HAL], a large public sector company. The company had an employee strength of over 25,000 and an enviable reputation as both a job-creating agency and, some said, an idler's paradise. For lack of work, many employees indulged in playing cards. This exaggerated account may not be entirely true, but it is true that in those days, unlike now, there were few takers except for the Air Force, whose planes were serviced by HAL.

Now HAL produces advanced fighter jets and has entered service contracts with the likes of Boeing and Airbus. A complete turnaround in its fortunes.

To look after the employees and their families located in different parts of the ever-expanding city, the company had a scheme of zonal medical officers. I was one of them and my area of practice also was close to their hospital. Though the monthly retainer fee was small, it was a welcome addition to my income. This job had its disadvantages and after many years I gave it up.

Normally, a regular patient sees me only when he or she was ill enough to warrant my attention. Minor ailments, coughs, and colds were either ignored or treated by using old prescriptions for similar ailments in the past. Even for routine follow-ups for chronic diseases like diabetes, I found my regular patients defaulting.

This was not so with these zonal patients. The patient and his or her family would come to seek my help for any and every sundry complaint for which a paying one would never come. Worse still was the person who wanted a sick leave certificate. Unverifiable complaints like headache, body aches, tiredness, loose bowels, and stomach pain were the usual complaints for which certificates were sought and sometimes reluctantly given.

Our Belliappa was one of these. He lived close by, and his house was a kilometre away from my practice premises. So, for him and his family, it was an easy walk. His wife, Seethamma, was an asthmatic and frequently needed to see me.

Belliappa suffered from chronic backache for which all kinds of investigations and tests available then had been done and a variety of medications given but his backache remained. It waxed and waned, and Belliappa attributed this to the full moon and the new moon. He felt better nearing a full moon and worse nearing a new moon. He was a firm believer in astrology.

Despite this, he came at least once a week, and sometimes I felt it was more to have a chat than for any medical help. He also had some faith and confidence in me as I had taught him some back-stretching exercises that had done him some good though they did not completely cure him. Also, I was able to control his wife's asthma, and her acute attacks had become much less frequent since she had become my patient.

Except for an occasional visit to see his wife when she was having severe wheezing, Belliappa did not request a house visit. So, when the call came from him, it was a bit of a surprise.

The call went like this:

"Doctor, my backache has become worse since this morning, will you be able to see me at home?"

I asked him, "Why don't you come see me now here?", meaning my clinic.

He said he felt too weak to walk and added that the backache had moved up and was now between his shoulder blades.

"Can it wait until I finish seeing patients and come in, say an hour from now?"

He said, "No problem, Doctor; take your time."

Though he told me to take my time, I was worried about his backache moving up and his weakness. I decided to go and see him immediately. Requesting my patients to wait, I took my bag and rushed to his house on my motorbike.

Seethamma opened the door and was surprised to see me as Belliappa had told her that I would come an hour later. I went to his room and found him sitting up, obviously in some discomfort, and also coughing. On examination, I found his pulse racing, his blood pressure low, and his lungs congested.

Our friend Belliappa had a heart attack and needed urgent admission. Getting an ambulance would take time, so I asked if anyone nearby had a car. The neighbour had one and I sent Seethamma to get on with this errand.

Belliappa asked, "Doctor, why don't you give me some injection? I will be better by evening, and then I will go."

I asked him, "How?"

"By scooter," he said.

I knew he was not aware of the seriousness of his condition and explained to him, in mild terms, why it was necessary to go to the hospital urgently.

The good neighbour arrived with his car. By then I had given Belliappa an injection of *Lasix* to drain the fluid from his lungs.

Preparing to get him to the car, I wanted him to sit on a chair so that we could lift him to the car. Belliappa would have none of this. *Was he not a brave Kodava?* He stood up, took a few steps, and collapsed.

We carried him to the HAL hospital three kilometres away. He was still alive, though barely conscious. Expert attention was given, and his heart attack was confirmed. He made a surprising recovery, considering the extent of the damage and his going into heart failure. Belliappa lived ten more years and died due to yet another heart attack.

✦✦◆✦

3
TOUCHING TALES

It was not Cataract: A Moving Experience

They were visiting the city because Mr. Suchit Nair's parents had settled here after retirement. They were my patients. Both Suchit and Priya were working in England and would have left after spending the next two weeks but for this incident.

The previous evening, the family had sat outside on the lawn. As I have written before, this extension was then mostly swamp, with hordes of mosquitoes attacking one come evening. Despite taking some anti-mosquito measures, the family had its own share of bites, which included the baby in the pram. Let me call this boy baby, Tharun. What follows is essentially his story:

The mosquito-bitten child developed a kind of redness around each bite and he was very uncomfortable. He was brought to me to have a look at these bites. While I was examining the restless child, I noticed that his eyes were not focusing, and his left eye had a whitish-yellow flare. This was distinctly abnormal, and I thought it could be a kind of congenital cataract. The bite allergy treatment became less important with this finding. The little fellow needed an urgent ophthalmology consultation.

Brigadier Krishnamurthy, after his retirement as an ophthalmology advisor to the armed forces, had settled in the present-day Defence Colony. He had converted a small part

109

of his home into an eye clinic and was my consultant for any eye issue I was faced with.

I took the parents and the child to him the same forenoon.

Brigadier had one look at the baby and told me, "Chidambar [my first name], this is not a cataract. It is much more serious. He has *retinoblastoma*, a kind of malignant tumour arising from the retina located at the back of the eyeball. This boy needs urgent surgery". This he told me in confidence.

I broke the bad news to the young couple and told them about the need for urgent intervention. The shocked couple decided to cut short their holidays and headed back to the UK.

Later I came to know that the eye with the tumour was removed. They found the other eye was involved too, and this was treated with radiation. The boy retained some vision, and when they visited here after some years, he could go about but with some difficulty. A few years later he went completely blind.

Tharun became a proficient piano player, played football, did his Ph.D. in chemistry, and taught that subject at the university level. This despite his blindness!

Patients who recover from retinoblastoma are prone to other types of cancer, and Tharun died last year, possibly due to some other type of cancer, and I had no heart to ask for the details.

Thus ended the remarkable story of a severely handicapped person, who overcame many odds and made a success of his short life.

Both parents live in the UK.

❖❖◆❖

The Power of Parental Love

Some fifteen years ago, while sitting in the foyer of the clubhouse, I noticed her. She looked familiar—a thin figure with the pinched face and hurried gait. I went across and accosted her. She was indeed who I thought she was. Fifteen years had passed, and she said I was often in her thoughts. It was the same with me.

When I first saw her daughter, the girl was just over two years old. A delightful little toddler she was, but prone to unexplained temper tantrums. The parents and I were at our wits' end to understand why. There was some suggestion that it could be a form of autism, but I found it hard to believe.

I found out the cause more by accident than by design. One day after the consult, I called out her name but got no response. I turned her around and got a nice smile and response. The ENT [ear-nose-throat] doctor attributed the delayed speech to normal development, and the parents were reassured that all would be well.

Now I was not so sure. The girl was born deaf, and we had not recognised it in time. Had we done so, even in those times, a cochlear implant could have been attempted. I spent time with the child and parents, and once we understood her problems, our attitude towards her changed. Her tantrums lessened and disappeared within the next two years.

Today, routine screening of newborns is done in major institutions, and cochlear implants have also become common, which, if done early, restore hearing to near normal.

What followed is worth recording. The father changed his job to one that gave him more time to spend with his daughter. The mother [the lady mentioned above] gave up her job to spend all her time with her daughter. They did a lot of research on deafness [I too learnt a lot from them] and on how to manage a deaf child. Both learnt sign language and how to teach phonation. They also decided not to have any more children. The mother showed enormous strength of character and courage, and after tiding over the crisis, she started working again.

Their sacrifice and effort paid off. The girl is now a normal seventeen-year-old pursuing her studies at a boarding school!

Real-life experiences like this are what I cherish. Nothing else in life gives me this kind of satisfaction and pleasure.

✧✧◆✧✧

The Heart of the Matter

Santosh, who passed away on January 11, 2025, was seventy years old, and his wife, Shireen, is a year younger. When I first met Santosh, he was seventeen, just out of school. His father was recovering from a heart attack. His father, Mr. V. G. Nedungadi, was in all sorts of financial trouble at that time due to the labour unrest in his factory, which he had been forced to close. These worries, combined with his pre-existing ischaemic heart disease, made him susceptible to the heart trouble he was then experiencing.

When Santosh met with me, it was to ask me to make a house call to see his father, who was not doing well post-heart attack. The family was then living in a large house on Ramakrishnappa Road in present-day Sarvagnanagar, then known as Cox Town. We old-timers still use that name.

That is how I met senior Nedungadi, a fine gentleman with old-world charm. He lived for twenty-six more years under my care and passed away in my presence at his home approximately thirty years ago.

The family had their own doctor. His name was Rama Rao, whose practice I had taken over after his death. The family at that time had no family doctor and probably wanted to try me out.

I must tell you briefly about Dr. Rama Rao, whose practice I had then acquired. I did not have the privilege of meeting Dr. Rama Rao but have heard stories about him from his patients, who became my patients after his death. The Nedungadi family too spoke highly of this doctor. Apparently, he never asked his patients for his fee but took whatever they gave him. Obviously, it was not enough. He supplemented this inadequate income by working part-time as an anaesthetist. He would go to the two or three nursing homes that existed in the city to administer anaesthesia and earn some money.

I realised that this also was not all that good when I visited his widow at the house where they lived—a very commonplace, lower-middle-class dwelling. I paid a princely sum of 3,000 rupees for his practice premises, which had some rickety furniture that had seen better days. I had to spend some additional amount to get the place into some sort of operational shape. Suffice it to say, I too came under some financial burden because of this venture.

Except for a few patients like Mr. Nedungadi, Dr. Rama Rao's practice consisted mainly of poor patients or those who acted as if they were, as I later discovered. Quite a few were freebooters and pay-later types.

The house call to see Mr. Nedungadi went well, and I met Santosh's mother and his still-to-be-married sister. Later, I met his US-based brother and sister. Over time, all of them became my patients.

Senior Nedungadi's precarious health and the stress of managing his factory and business led young Santosh, just out of school, to take over and run the family business. The years between seventeen and twenty-five were busy ones for him, filled with activities such as participation in theatre and drama, Rotary, and running the inherited business.

His involvement in amateur theatre led him to meet Shireen, also a passionate theatre enthusiast. Their friendship gradually blossomed into love.

Santosh had gone to Madras [now Chennai] on a business errand and developed severe vomiting and chest discomfort. He called me to ask for advice. He also read out the prescription from the doctor he had seen there. Even to this day, I don't know why I urged him to return to Bangalore immediately—intuition, perhaps?

He returned on the next flight and stopped by to see me on his way from the airport [which was then just fifteen minutes away from my place]. I examined him and found his BP a bit low with some missed beats. An urgent ECG revealed a recent inferior wall infarction. At the young age of twenty-five, Santosh had suffered a heart attack. I admitted him to a hospital, and after two weeks, he made an uneventful recovery. A modified TMT [Treadmill Test] showed no fresh changes.

Thus began a lifelong follow-up and drastic lifestyle change, which he continued to follow for the next forty-five years. His high blood pressure, diabetes, and heart disease remained well-controlled. He is a testament to what can be achieved with regular exercise, diet, and weight control, in addition to medication and regular physician follow-ups, even with a poor family history and co-morbid conditions such as diabetes and high blood pressure.

When he was in the hospital recovering from the heart attack, Shireen came to see me. She asked, "Doc, how serious is Santosh's condition?"

"Stable," I said.

"How long is he going to live?" was her next question.

This was a difficult question to answer. I don't recall what exactly I told her, but I distinctly remember her reply.

She said, "Five years of quality life is good enough for me; we will go ahead and get married."

So, they did.

Shireen's mother was Hindu, and her father was Muslim. Based on what I know of Shireen and her sisters, they must have had a reasonably liberal upbringing.

Their marriage lasted forty years and resulted in two children, both of whom are married and well-settled in the United States. All of them remain my patients to this day.

(The family's consent was secured to share this narrative.)

❖❖◆❖

A Bond Beyond the Clinic

His name was Madhavan Nayar. I must reassure my other two patients, Madhavan Nayars, who are alive and kicking, that this is a pseudonym.

It must have been thirty years since I had known him and, as often happens with us general practitioners, initially as a patient and over the years also as a friend. Now, looking at him lying in dishevelled clothes in a badly-made bed, made me think not of the indignity of death but of the *peculiar personality* of Mr. Nayar and what drew us to each other.

I keep a tidy examination room with a fresh white sheet spread over the examination couch each day, and sometimes twice a day. Despite this, there would be a few discernible smudges, especially at the foot end of the sheet.

No one minded this until I met Mr. Madhavan Nayar. When his turn came to be examined, he took one quick look at the table, politely excused himself, said he would return in the evening if I did not mind, and went away.

115

When he returned in the evening, he had a small bag with him. From this bag, he took out a clean white sheet and proceeded to spread it on my examination couch, all the while apologising for his action and requesting me not to be offended. I was not offended, having met many with much stranger personalities than this one. After the examination was over, he neatly folded the sheet and put it back in his bag.

That is how we met. Since then, each time he visited me, he followed this procedure. This fastidious nature was in keeping with the general character of the man. He was one of my few patients who always telephoned me before coming, despite knowing that I did not follow the appointment system in those days. He was always on time, even if it meant waiting for his turn.

Since we lived in the same area and belonged to the same club, we also had the same barber. On one occasion, I bumped into him as he was coming out of the barber's shop. His usual bag was with him, and I, *of course*, knew what it contained.

When I went in, I asked the barber about the bag. Like other members of his trade, this one too loved telling a story. Not only did Mr. Nayar have a white sheet for his exclusive use but also a whole range of barbering equipment, well-packed in a special case, down to the last *new blade*. He made the barber wash his hands and dip them in a solution of disinfectant before allowing him to touch his head.

When I heard this, I wondered why he did not make me wash my hands before examining him. Maybe he had observed me washing my hands after examining each patient and therefore did not feel the need. But I certainly do not dip my hands in disinfectant. I wondered then when he would make this request of me, and if he did, what I should do!

We met occasionally at the club over drinks. His order was precise: a small whisky of a specific brand, two ice cubes, and an equal amount of water. The ice cubes were to go into the glass first. When the glass with whisky arrived, he would hold it up to the light and give it a close look to see if there were any fingerprints. If he found any, the order would be repeated. The waiters were wise to his ways, and his glass was always well-wiped before the drink was poured.

I would often wonder whether he was an obsessive-compulsive. Even if he was, no one was unhappy, least of all Mrs. Nayar. He had a very happy family life and a close circle of friends who liked him. He was also a very successful businessman.

But in death, he was like anyone else. After the certification formalities were over, I asked his son to get me his shaving kit. We gave him a good shave, taking care to use a *new blade*. We dressed him in a new shirt and a *mundu* and spread a clean sheet over him after replacing the old bed sheet with a new one.

With that done, I thought he was ready to receive the mourning friends and relatives in his accustomed style.

I returned home with mixed feelings: a sense of sorrow for having lost a friend and a sense of satisfaction for having done something for him. This, I am sure, he would have appreciated had he been alive.

✧✧✧✧

Doctor's Dues

When I began my practice some fifty-five years back, my area [the present-day Indiranagar] was underdeveloped, with three big villages dominating the fledgling extension. There was one eatery called Durga Bhavan. This eatery was the only reasonably well-maintained place and had good custom. The owner was one Ram Udupa, who hailed from a village near Kundapura and naturally made friends with me. He consulted

117

with me whenever there were any health issues with his staff or with his family.

He looked after his employees well but also knew how to extract work. He had many attributes of a successful businessman. One of them was that whenever he brought an employee to me, he would pay the fee but would make the employee hand over the money to me.

The ploy was successful in that I charged a fee that was much less than usual, as I knew he would deduct this from the salary he paid at the end of the month. I probably would have charged more had he paid directly without the employee's knowledge. This was the scenario when Ram Udupa brought his employee Ganesh Karantha to see me.

Very thin, bordering on what could be called emaciation, undernourished, tottering, needing support even to walk, obviously very sick, the young man came in. One look at him, and I knew he was very ill. I made him lie down and proceeded to examine him.

He had a festering wound on his foot [the result of a food-laden plate falling on his foot some ten days back] with swelling all around and a painful swelling in his groin area. He was also running a high fever. All were signs and symptoms of the spread of infection in his bloodstream. Strictly speaking, he needed urgent attention, preferably in a hospital.

I told Mr. Udupa the seriousness of the issue. He said, "Doctor, you do your best. He, you can see, is a poor boy from my native village who has studied up to SSLC [Secondary School Leaving Certificate] and taking him to the hospital means a lot of trouble to everyone. We are short-handed as it is; we will see how it goes for a couple of days."

Those were the days when penicillin worked like magic in such cases. I removed all the muck around the wound, cleaned it, placed a clean bandage, and asked him to be brought daily for a penicillin injection.

He did not turn up the next day. I found out he could not walk, and there was no escort to bring him. Everyone was busy. After finishing my morning work, I went to the hotel with my bag to see him. Ram Udupa was happy to see me and took me to see the boy at the back of the hotel.

There I was exposed to the pathetic living conditions of these workers: a single room shared by four people, poorly ventilated, and with a bathroom outside. Not an ideal place to live, but that was the best the owner could do. The patient was not worse and appeared a bit better and was able to eat food that morning. I changed his dressing and gave him another shot of penicillin. I repeated the procedure the third day too. The fourth day, Ganesha came to the clinic after walking two kilometres and said he felt much better.

It took two more injections and ten more days for the wound to heal and for him to become normal. The groin swelling too disappeared.

At the end of the month, he appeared.

I asked him, "What is the matter now?"

He said he had come to pay my fee. I was taken aback. Here was a poor man who wanted to pay my fee. I told him I would take it from Mr. Ram Udupa, his boss. He did not appear pleased. After I insisted, he reluctantly went. This youngster, who was getting a hundred rupees per month as his wage, of which he must have sent some to his people at home, wanted to pay me.

The next visit was when he was sick with an attack of asthma. In those days, especially at the onset of rain, many people suffered from severe cases of asthma. Unlike these days, we did not have inhaled medications and relied on adrenaline to treat acute attacks, along with a dose of injectable steroid thrown in for good measure. This was followed by oral medications for long-term use. These oral drugs had many side effects like a racing heart, stomach irritation, *etc.* But then that was the best we could do fifty years ago.

Then the city of Bangalore could be called the 'asthma city' of India, especially the outlying extensions like where I lived, then named Binnamangala before it got the glamorous name of Indiranagar. This Binnamangala had many low-lying swampy areas full of parthenium weed, popularly called congress grass [ragweed in the United States].

This noxious weed arrived in India along with the gift of wheat from the United States to tide over our food crisis in the fifties. It had no natural enemies, could not be used as fodder, and it bred and bred and spewed millions of spores into the atmosphere. These spores were highly allergic and made asthma even worse.

Our Karantha was a victim. The usual dose of injection of adrenaline with steroids soon made him feel better, and he left, taking the prescription for long-term use.

I did not hear or see him for months. When asked, Ram Udupa had a one-word answer, "That boy is not cut out for the hotel waiter's job," meaning thereby that Karantha was not working for him anymore.

Karantha came nearly a year later, this time again for repeated attacks of asthma. He looked better and more self-confident. He showed me the prescriptions of some city-based doctors. I asked him why he did not come to see me. "Because you do not take your fee," he answered.

I promised him I would keep an account of his taking help from me hereafter, and he could pay me when his financial position improved. This appeared to please him somewhat, and he left after taking my prescription. He came several times in the next two years, and then came a period when I did not see him for five years. I occasionally wondered what could have happened to him.

One fine morning, after a lapse of five years, he came to see me. At first, I could not recognise him. He had put on weight, looked and behaved with much more confidence, and was well-dressed. I asked him his whereabouts and why he was away for so long.

He said, "I finished my PUC while working in another hotel in the city whose owner allowed me to attend evening classes. Then I took a part-time job, finished my BCom, and got a rank. I have passed the All-India Banking Services Examination, and I needed to visit Bangalore for training before I get posted."

"And I have to also clear your dues," he added and stopped.

"What dues? I have not kept any account," I said.

"But you said you would," he pressed.

I told him he had more than made up for not paying my fee. He would not take no for an answer, took an envelope from his pocket, placed it on my table, and took his leave.

Before leaving, he told me he was presently living in Hubli. I used to hear from him occasionally. As it happens, distance, both physical and geographical, often makes us lose contact. I thus lost track of this remarkable young man.

❖❖◆❖

ESR-iously Speaking

We doctors order investigations when we are stumped as to what is wrong with the patient or sometimes to know the effect of a treatment. We also order tests to assess fitness levels. This last phenomenon, which was exceptional when I began my career, has now become routine. It is so common that patients themselves go to the laboratory, get tests done, and then see us. Most often it is a sheer waste of money but occasionally it results in early diagnosis and effective management.

When tests are ordered, a common one among them is called the ESR. ESR stands for erythrocyte sedimentation rate. In simple language, it means the speed with which the red cells of the blood drop when a column of blood is suspended in a glass tube. This simple screening test is very nonspecific. It tells us that there is something wrong but does not tell us where and what is wrong. A friend of mine joked that even a few hard sneezes could elevate the ESR.

Red blood cells are far more numerous than white blood cells. Their main purpose is to carry oxygen to the tissues. Normally, they circulate without clumping, and when suspended, they settle very slowly. In disease conditions, the rate of this fall is rapid. The higher the fall, the more serious the disease.

We accumulate, *willy-nilly*, a lot of unwanted material in the blood during our lives. These include, among other things, bacterial and viral antigens, against which the immune system produces antibodies, and particulate materials that circulate in our blood. The amounts of these materials often exceed the capacity of our innate cleaning systems. Some of these stick to the surface of the cells and make them not only heavy but also get them to stick to one another. The once-clean cells become laden with debris and heavy, thus settling faster in suspension, causing the ESR to rise. In acute infections and malignancies, this phenomenon is marked. And very high ESR levels are always worrying to the attending doctor.

Mrs. R, a fifty-year-old woman, was with a group of friends when one of them told her that she looked pale. Everyone looks pale in artificial light, and Mrs. R did not attach any importance to this comment. A few days later, another friend said, "What is the matter with you? You are looking very

122

pale." Similar remarks on two subsequent occasions made her worried.

She decided to get the tests done. Had she come to me, I probably would have examined her and, more likely than not, not ordered any tests. She went to a well-known lab and told the receptionist that she wanted tests for her paleness. Most labs are privately owned, and clients like Mrs. R are like a new lode of gold for them. All tests, including scans of her chest and abdomen, were performed.

Here is something interesting. It is not difficult to find some trivial abnormality in most people, and as they say [half in jest], "When you see a tail sticking out of a hole, it is sometimes best not to pull it out, as you don't know whether you will pull out a cat or a leopard." Labs, too, have a similar way of reporting. They place an asterisk against the slightest abnormality. In Mrs. R's case, there were many such asterisks!

Thoroughly frightened, Mrs. R landed in my clinic with a whole wad of papers. "I am very sick," she said by the way of opening remark. She looked very fit, and I said so.

"No, no, you see these reports and then you will change your opinion," she said. As she insisted that she was very sick, I felt I should examine her before reviewing her papers. She agreed, and a ten-minute physical found her to be in good condition, with her basic vital parameters being normal.

Now came the time to see her lab reports and scan reports. I could see her becoming visibly anxious. Almost all her reports, including the ones marked with an asterisk, were normal. However, there was one major abnormality. Her ESR was very high. Normally, in her age group, the ESR should not exceed 20 mm/hour; hers was 80.

This was indeed a surprise and a cause for worry. I was surprised because she appeared healthy, and I could find no explanation for the high ESR. In the absence of infection, the only other cause could be *occult* [hidden cancer]. In women, the most likely place is the breast where small tumours could easily be missed. I felt her breasts once again. I could find no mass, small or big. I found among her papers recent tests excluding cervical [uterine] and ovarian cancer. Then where was it? Could this be in her blood-forming bone marrow? Could this be in her colon? Or lungs?

I had no option but to get a whole lot of expensive tests done. Maybe a better option would be to send her to an institution [an unsettling thought]. My brain was buzzing with all sorts of thoughts as I was leafing through her papers and saw her liver function test reports. There was a marginal increase in the globulin fraction of her blood protein. Globulins are very important components of our immune system and special cells called plasma cells make these.

Here was a possible clue. Without telling her what I was thinking but reassuring her nonetheless, I ordered a test called serum protein electrophoresis, in which the various fractions of blood proteins are studied in a non-invasive test. She returned two days later with the report. She had a raised level of one particular fraction of her gamma globulin.

I, at last, had the diagnosis: monoclonal gammopathy of uncertain significance [MGUS]. This condition is due to the excessive production of one type of gamma globulin by a single clone of cells. This excess protein adheres to the surface of the red blood cells, thus making them heavier and causing them to settle faster in suspension.

Monoclonal gammopathy is a premalignant condition, and over time, a percentage of those affected with this develop a type of cancer called multiple myeloma. No one knows who will progress to this serious condition and who will not. I have had several patients who carried MGUS to their grave without developing multiple myeloma.

I painted the picture, highlighting the positive aspects. That was ten years ago. She is now seventy. The other day, she had come for her usual follow-up with her reports. They were all normal, and she, too, will hopefully carry this condition to her grave without developing cancer, whenever her time comes.

Postscript:

The patient in question, Mrs. Rajani Seroo, underwent further workup both here and in Mumbai. Her illness was diagnosed as *Waldenström's macroglobulinemia*, a condition characterised by an increase in the globulin fraction of the blood proteins. This is a slow-growing type of lymphoma arising from B lymphocytes, which are precursors of plasma cells.

Mrs. Rajani, along with her son Saurabh, founded the first Waldenström's macroglobulinemia support group in India, called *Waldenstrom India* in 2019. This support group has helped numerous patients with similar conditions and their caregivers by providing information on managing the disease and where to seek help.

You can access the website at http://www.wmindia.org

❖❖❖❖

The Big House, the Hidden Hurt

This is another story from the past. Forty-five years ago, when this lady and her family became my patients, this area [Indiranagar, Bangalore], which is now considered a posh upmarket locality, was ill-served even with basic civic amenities. The roads were ill-lit and badly surfaced. Commuting to the city was tough, with very few buses serving the extension. Shopping was limited to a few poorly stocked stores. There were a few villages around, though, which had existed probably for centuries, and my clinic was one of the very few which provided basic medical services.

The lady whose story I am telling here is now past seventy years. When I first met her, she was a strapping, fecund woman in her late twenties, happily producing children [she ended up having six boys and one girl]. The first encounter was a house call that ended as a surgical emergency, diagnosed in fading light one grimy, rainy night with no facility even for a proper examination. The clinical diagnosis of gallbladder infection proved correct, and a surgical removal of her gallbladder cured her.

This episode made her my patient and later my friend for life. Except for her husband, the whole family, and later even her grandchildren became my patients. The family has done well financially over the years.

In addition to the ravages of age, she has developed hypertension, a leaking aortic [heart] valve, severe diabetes with neuropathy, and seasonal bronchial asthma. Needless to say, her visits to me have become more frequent now than before.

When she visited me some months ago, she was not looking good and after the consultation was over, she said very diffidently, "Doctor, I will not be able to pay your fee," and then broke down with fits of huge sobs. I keep quiet in such situations and allow the person to finish crying. I have learnt that they all eventually come out with what they have come to say, and then it is easy to manage.

After a while, she wiped her tears and said, "My husband says I spend too much money on doctors and visits to the hospitals and it is better that I die."

This took me by surprise. Here is a wealthy family that lived in a big house with assistants, a cook, two cars with drivers, and an ongoing, flourishing business. And this woman, the lady of the house, has been told to die because her medical

126

expenses are unaffordable. Surely there is some mistake somewhere. I told her as much.

She said, "Doctor, you don't know the truth. What I have had to put up in the last fifty years with that man! Never was there a day he has asked me what I wanted or how I was doing; even now, my illness is an irritant to him, and he really feels that I should die, as I have lived beyond my utility to him and his children."

I said a few words of sympathy and told her to come as long as she wanted to and not to worry about paying.

That proud woman has not turned up since then. I don't know what happened to her, as the family no longer comes to me.

✧✧◆✧

4

BEYOND ILLNESS

Usman Khan's Gift: A Meat-y Surprise

I have on an earlier occasion written about Usman Khan and
his diet. I have also mentioned how I came to know him and
his becoming my patient. When he became my patient, his
family was small and remained small, thanks to my advice on
family planning, which the couple followed meticulously. This
and other matters related to his and his relative's health,
which I took care of, drew us close, and I was the recipient of
a discount whenever I went to his fruit shop in Shivajinagar
market.

The day was Eid, an important festival for Muslims. I was just
about to close the clinic and there arrived Usman and his
family resplendent in new clothes and happiness writ large on
their faces. Obviously, they had not come seeking help for
any illness; it was just to wish me and leave.

If it was just that, there would not have been any problem.
But what followed was something which I vividly remember
to this day.

I wished all of them *Eid Mubarak* and asked what they were
up to. Rehana [Usman's wife] said they were planning to go
to Cubbon Park and then, for the evening, eat out.

Now it was Usman's turn. He slowly took out from his bag a
nicely wrapped packet and a small bag of fruits, placed these
on my table, and said in chaste Urdu, "I have brought it,
especially for you. It is quite fresh; please don't refuse."

He gave me no option. I accepted it with thanks, and the happy family left for their outing.

The fruits appeared fresh, but what was the other fresh item inside the wrapped packet? I slowly opened it, and to my *horror and surprise*, it contained a large piece of mutton, obviously freshly cut!

I am by choice a vegetarian, and my family are compulsive ones. I just could not take this horror of a gift [from my family's perspective] home.

I drove to Mr. Robert D'Souza's house and handed over the gift to him. Robert and Lizzy are good friends of mine. Lizzy did most of my secretarial work for free, and I, in turn, looked after them. Robert was ecstatic to see the gift.

He said, "Doctor, it is rare that we get such tender and fresh meat. Many thanks to you and your friend." He did not stop there but continued, "What about that fruit bag? Isn't it contaminated? It has kept company in your scooter's dicky. Why not leave it here?"

I did not have an apt answer to this impertinence. I went home with fruit bag, minus the mutton wrap, and it was very welcome.

Now comes the question of how Usman presumed that I and my family are meat eaters? The culprit was my neighbour Ghouse who had a cloth and tailoring business. This Ghouse and Usman were friends. And Usman was told by this Mr. *know-it-all* Ghouse that the Doctor [me] is from the army, and in the army, everyone eats meat, as otherwise they cannot survive. So, he told Usman to give me the present. This was told to me by Usman some months later.

For successive Eids, he has confined himself to giving me fruits as gifts.

❖❖◆❖❖

Resurrection
(Written some years back)

My friend, the late Dr. Prabhakar, was a busy practitioner in the inner city. Like many other GPs [General Practitioners] with busy practices, he too found it difficult to make house calls during his clinic hours, which often extended to late nights.

When the call came requesting an urgent visit to see an elderly patient, it was 7 pm and the clinic was full of patients. There was no way he could get out leaving them waiting as the caller lived five kilometres away, and going by the dense traffic, it would be at least two hours before he would return.

He however couldn't refuse the call either, as the patient was an old family friend and suffered from diabetes and heart disease. He told the caller, who was the patient's eldest son, that he would try to make the house call around 10 pm and that if the patient's condition was very serious, he should shift his father to a nearby hospital and let him know.

At 8 pm another call came informing that the night visit was no longer required as the patient had breathed his last.

This occasionally happens to us GPs because, despite advice, patients refuse to go and seek help elsewhere and sometimes pay a heavy price. Dr. Prabhakar was now a very unhappy man with many troubling thoughts in his head. Had he gone, leaving his clinic when the call came, would the patient have survived? Had he failed to assess the seriousness of the call? Should he have insisted that they take the patient to the hospital? He was filled with guilt and remorse. These feelings torment us for weeks and months and form an unpleasant part of a GP's life.

A shaken Dr. Prabhakar did not sleep well that night. Early the next morning, he went to the house of the deceased with the intention of offering his condolences to the bereaved family and to issue a death certificate. Normally, the atmosphere in and around the house where a death has occurred is sombre and sad. That this is often contrived is a different matter.

One would see groups of friends and relations of the deceased huddled and engaged in hushed conversation with grave looks on their faces. Amongst most Hindu families there would also be a small earthen pot filled with burning wood emitting smoke, a sure signal to all and sundry that a death has occurred in that home, and you are at liberty to take a breather and gawk.

To the Doctor's surprise and some consternation, none of these were visible outside the house. For a moment, he thought that the body had already been taken away and the mourners had left. But who could have issued the death certificate, without which the body cannot be cremated? Could it be that another doctor was called to attend to the deceased? Had that doctor issued the certificate? This assumption made him feel a bit better.

These were his thoughts when he pressed the doorbell.

After a while, the door opened and the old man who was supposed to be dead was standing in front with a wide grin on his face. It was a shock and made my friend take a step back!

After a few seconds, when there was no speech from either party, the old man's son arrived on the scene and narrated the following story:

"After I called you, I went back to see my father. He was restless and breathing very hard and moving his hands as though to tell me something. After a few minutes, he stopped breathing, and his arms and legs became still, and he closed his eyes. I thought he had died, so I called you to tell you not to come and also informed the relatives and friends of his death.

132

"Within the next half an hour people started coming, and one by one they started pouring spoonfuls of milk into his mouth, as is our custom. This went on for some time, and suddenly we noticed *it* [he pointed towards his father] moving the legs and making noises. This made the relatives scatter in a hurry. I too was frightened.

"A little later, my father slowly got up and looked around and asked, 'What are all these people doing?' He also said he felt very hungry. We fed him and told him what had happened."

"Father has not stopped abusing me since then," added the son, looking appropriately contrite.

The old man was a diabetic, had missed his lunch, and had barely eaten in the evening. He had taken his insulin shot later than usual that day and had gone into a coma induced by low blood sugar. Mistakenly believing him to be dead, the family poured milk into his mouth, which revived him!

The old man lived for another five years and did not have any repeat episodes, and when he eventually died, it was a *dead cert*.

❖❖❖❖❖

Lost and Found

It was the persistent whimper that drew my attention. It appeared to be a child's small but persistent cry. I went out to the waiting area to investigate. The waiting room was empty but for this two-year-old who was sitting on the floor weeping.

In my clinic, I am not only the doctor but also the cook, the babysitter, and the bottle washer. I don't have a receptionist or help to manage the patients and take calls. I have, over the years, trained my patients to be disciplined and take their turn, and I take the calls myself.

133

Though many of my friends have found managing a practice without help tough, I have found it better this way as long as I don't perform procedures that need assistance. So don't wonder how the consulting area was so empty. But for this little fellow, there was *not a soul* in sight.

Seeing me he brightened up and stopped crying but that did not solve my problem. Where did he come from? None of my neighbours had a toddler of this age and he couldn't have trespassed into my clinic from the road. The wild thought that someone had intentionally abandoned this boy in my clinic was dismissed as unreasonable.

The only conclusion that I could come to was that the couple who came in last, which was a good half an hour ago, must have forgotten the boy and left. Though that was the only possible explanation, I couldn't understand how one can *forget a child* who is with you, leave him, and go!

Then, was he there when they came out? Was it possible that the mother made him sit outside and came in to see me and this boy went outside to investigate my little garden around the house and was not there when the parents came out after the consultation?

Yes, that seemed likely. I asked the boy with gestures if he had gone out. He replied in Malayalam [and his Malayalam vocabulary was better than mine], and what he told me was that he needed his mother. This answer was followed by another bout of crying, this time louder.

I picked him up and tried to comfort him by telling him that his mother would soon be here. His cry was even louder, as obviously he did not follow what I said, or he had no confidence in me.

I thought some bribery would help. So, I took him inside and gave him a piece of chocolate. He stopped crying and was occupied with gobbling up the sweet for the next few minutes. The job done, he became restless again and began asking for his mother.

I took him out and stood near the gate. My curious neighbour who was passing by asked me, "So, Doctor, at last, you have a grandson?" [He knew I am too old to have a son of this age]. I had to tell him why and how this little boy was not my grandson.

"If the mother doesn't turn up, he will be *yours*," was his parting and rather uncharitable remark.

We went inside, and by now we had become friends. The boy was not demanding his mother, having probably found a better alternative who gave him an endless supply of sweets and did not mind playing with him. My worries too faded as I was busy with him.

Things thus stood when I heard a loud commotion outside. That was the return of the mother. She had at last realised that her son was found safe and sound.

As I had thought, when she came out, the boy was not sitting where she had parked him but was out in the garden, possibly not visible. She was so preoccupied with discussing her problem with her husband that both of them forgot about the boy. Stranger was the fact that from my clinic they had gone to the chemist's and then had driven home. Only when they reached home did they realise that their child was missing. It took some time for them to deduce that he must be with me.

It was a relief to all concerned to see this reunion!

That was the first and the last time a child was left behind. Other objects that have been found unattended include umbrellas, ladies' bags and purses, shawls, briefcases, mobile phones, footwear, spectacles, a drunk patient and once even a *dead patient.*

❖❖❖❖

The Sheikh's Generous Gesture

Some forty years ago, this city was small, and there weren't many large hospitals. There was a distinct separation between the city and the cantonment, and Muslims formed a sizeable portion of the population residing in the cantonment area. There was a small nursing home in this area where my friend, Dr. Chandra, worked as a surgeon. The incident narrated below was told to me by this friend.

One afternoon when the crowd of outpatients was sparse and the receptionist was not too busy, she was rudely shaken by the guard at the gate, who came inside looking panic-stricken. He said, "Madam, many cars full of *Arabbis* outside. All want to come inside."

Now the hapless receptionist went outside with the guard to find out what was happening. At the entrance, she found an Arab sheikh, three women, four children and a helper who was trying to translate what the sheikh was telling her. The women went inside and occupied whatever chairs that were vacant, and the children began using the portico and the small garden as their playground.

The *Dubhashi* [translator] translated in bad Urdu, what the sheikh was saying. First, he confirmed that they had come to the right place and had not mistaken it for a hotel, as the receptionist had first thought. Then he said, "This Sheikh Sulaiman, following a recommendation from his Indian friend who is from this part of the city, has come here for treatment," and showed the letter that Sulaiman had written and the reply he had received from this hospital.

In that letter he had asked for twelve rooms!

Thoroughly confused, that poor receptionist called the resident doctor who also looked after the management, to come urgently to handle this emergency. That poor doctor who had just gone home, which was nearby, after a busy

136

morning's work, had to hurriedly get back to take stock of the situation.

When he saw the party, he too was surprised. He had thought that 'twelve rooms' was a typing mistake as no one would want twelve rooms for a single patient and replied that arrangements would be made for the surgery and recovery. It took more than an hour for him and a three-way conversation to convince the sheikh to move his harem and progeny to a nearby star hotel and to allot him the room reserved for him and another for his secretary-cum-interpreter.

A call went to my friend Dr. Chandra to come and see the patient that evening. When he went to see the patient with the nurse, the room was empty and so was the interpreter's. Neither of them was found inside, but their belongings were intact. Where had they gone? Calls were made to the hotel where the families were staying.

"Yes, they did come but have gone out some time back," said the wives, and they too were now anxious to know where these two had gone. By then it was seven in the evening, and Dr. Chandra went home after seeing his other patients.

It was around 10 pm that Sheikh Sulaiman and his interpreter friend returned to the nursing home to the relief of all concerned, including the family. Following the advice of his Dubai-based Indian friend, the duo had visited a bar-cum-restaurant and had a great time drinking and eating.

Basic tests were done the next day, and his surgery for removal of the swelling on his back was duly done.

The day of discharge arrived, and Sulaiman sent word to Dr. Chandra that he wanted to meet him one last time before leaving. Dr. Chandra went to see him. After profusely thanking him, Sulaiman handed over a beribboned gift package to the doctor, all the time profusely thanking him.

On returning home, Dr. Chandra found an expensive suit material along with a high-end shirt and a matching tie. There was also some cash to take care of the tailoring charges.

Dr. Chandra duly proceeded and got the suit made.

The nursing home celebrates its founding day, when all the staff, along with the doctors, are invited. Some entertainment, followed by fellowship and dinner. This is a much-awaited event when all those working at the nursing home get a chance to interact with one another.

Dr. Chandra went attired in his recently done suit with the matching shirt and tie. He found that most, if not all, had come wearing the same attire, which included the menial staff like the barber and the security guard!

Our Sulaiman was a true socialist. He did not differentiate between the chief surgeon and the lowly barber. All had received the same gift.

❖❖◆❖

Worry about Small Size

Rudrappa, when this episode happened, must have been about twenty-five years old and came from a second-generation educated family. His mother was a schoolteacher, and his father was in government service. I had known this family of four for five years or so and when I first saw Rudrappa [I called him Rudra] he was in college.

He rarely fell ill and kept good health but was withdrawn and difficult to communicate with, and his replies were always in monosyllables. It appeared as though he was having some ongoing mental health issues.

He came to see me one day. I congratulated him on getting a job so soon after his graduation.

I asked him the reason why he had come. He said rather reluctantly, "My that thing is very small." That thing meant his penis. This was not the first young man who had seen me with this complaint.

I asked him, "How do you know?"

"I have measured it," he said.

This was becoming interesting. The human penis in adults, when not erect, can be very small and can even be hidden in the folds of skin and when erect it can vary in size and length depending on the build and height of the man. It can be anywhere from four to seven inches. I asked him whether he had measured it in the erect or flaccid state. He said it was half an inch when quiet and four when erect.

I asked him, "Why are you worried?"

He said, "My marriage is fixed, and I may not be able to have sex if my penis is this small."

This misinformation came from his "expert" friends and some blue magazines he had read. In those days, there was no internet or Google search. I don't know what would have happened to Rudra if he had had access to these—worse, maybe.

The next half-hour was spent in convincing him that for his build and height, it was perfectly normal, and he was perfectly capable of satisfactory performance. And there was no need for any medication to increase his organ's size.

He left, apparently very satisfied.

Two weeks later, he came one morning looking ill and frightened. I asked him what had happened.

"Doctor, I did one big mistake," he said.

"What big mistake?" I asked.

"I went with my friend and visited a call girl [he used a different name] two days ago and am now having severe pain when I pee," he mumbled, looking down.

I examined him and found he had urethral discharge and pain. The sex worker had given him gonorrhoea in exchange for his attempt to prove his manhood. I counselled him about the dangers of having unprotected sex. After a couple of injections of penicillin, he got cured.

His marriage was successful, and he lived away from this city as his job in the border road organisation took him to different places. I lost touch with him and his family after some years.

❖❖◆❖❖

Machado and his Mother-in-Law

Stanley Machado, popularly known as Stan, is a sixty-year-old Gulf returnee. It was some twenty years ago, that I first met him and his wife Anna. At that time, both lived with Anna's mother, Beth, in the old Fraser Town [now Pulakeshinagar]. The large house was inherited by Beth and would go to her daughter Anna after she [Beth] passed away.

You might be wondering how Stan and Anna's family, with their children, came to live with the old lady after returning from the Gulf. This was a move of convenience, as the children were in school and college, and the old lady also needed someone to be with her. This happy state of affairs lasted for some five years or so, when the trouble began between the mother and the daughter.

Even the smallest issue would lead to verbal battles that dragged on for days, with Stan frequently called upon to referee. And he only complicated matters further, as the arguing parties accused him of taking sides, regardless of his actions.

Matters became so bad that Anna decided to move to her native town Mangalore where her eldest son Joseph had settled, leaving poor Stan to manage her mother and the big house. She would make a couple of quick visits to the city, say hello to both husband and mother, and make her quick departure before the mother would flare up.

This was the situation when the trouble with Beth began. She sent word for me to see her. When Stan came to pick me up, I asked him, "Stan, what is the problem with your mother-in-law?"

He said, "Will she ever confide in me about her problem? She just ordered me to get the doctor. That is all I know. Hope you will be able to find out what is wrong with her. To my eyes, the *old coot* looks as fit as ever."

I went to see her.

Beth was sitting in an armchair reading the day's newspaper. On seeing me she happily said good morning and told Stan, who was hovering around, to get lost.

After he left, she told me in a conspiratorial tone, "This son-in-law of mine is out to kill me."

This was news to me.

I told her, "Why do you think so? He is a nice man."

"Nice man to you maybe, but for me he is a *devil* with nice manners."

"How do you know he is trying to kill you?" I asked.

"The soup is tasting bitter, and I think he is adding arsenic to slowly kill me," was her reply.

To reassure her I said that there are many reasons for bitter taste and ageing is one of them.

"Doctor, you do not know; I have now started having ready-to-eat soup and not the one prepared at home, and it is

141

tasting normal. If he thinks he can kill me, he should think differently. I also have started carrying *this*." She showed me a pocketknife!

I asked her why she wanted to see me, and she said, "This tension is causing me to lose sleep. Can you give me some medicine to sleep?"

This was easy enough—to give a sedative and leave.

On the way back, I asked Stan jokingly, "Since when have you started doing this to your mother-in-law?"

He said, "Doc, that is another story. She began having this suspicion some three years back; I am not the only suspect, our cook and gardener also are. She has taken to locking her bedroom so that I will not be able to kill her at night."

I knew that the old lady had some form of dementia with delusions. Should I interfere or wait? I decided to wait.

Some months later there was another call from Beth. When she saw me, her opening remark was, "I told you last time that Stan is trying to kill me, you did not believe me. See now what has happened."

I asked her, "What has happened?"

She showed me a bowl that had some saliva-like liquid. I asked her, "What is this?"

She said, "Can't you see? It is full of blood; every time I cough, blood comes out. I got an X-ray done, and it says normal. Then why am I spitting blood, tell me? It is all my son-in-law's doing. I am planning to lodge a police complaint."

Now I was certain that Beth had Schizophrenia and needed urgent medication. How do I tell her? Even if I told her she would not believe me. I took the easy way out.

I asked her, "Are you taking the nighttime sleeping tablet?"

She said "Yes, but it is not helping me."

I had an opening now. I said, "I will add another medicine to help you to sleep better. I will also caution Stan. In the meantime, don't go to the police. It will do more harm than good." That seemed to mollify her a bit.

I added a drug called olanzapine to her existing sedative and returned home.

Four weeks later, Stan met with me. He said, "Doc, that new drug is wonderful. She has stopped accusing me, and this time, after many years, she did not pick up a fight with her daughter when she visited her. My wife is thinking of moving back to Bangalore. The only problem is, she is always hungry and sleeps all the time."

I asked him, "Is it not better to have a *sleepy and docile* mother-in-law than one who is aggressive and accuses her son-in-law of trying to kill her?"

His smile was the answer.

❖❖❖❖

A Gurkha's Love Story

When this happened, my colony was small and the roads were ill-lit. Petty thefts were not uncommon. The residents got together and employed a nightbeat named Dilbahadur. At that time, he must have been in his early twenties and this Gurkha had recently come from Nepal. He had a ready grin on his face and did his job with enthusiasm.

Sometimes I felt he overdid his nightbeat's job. He had a stout stick in his hand and was prone to using it to create a noise by banging on the road and on the gates of the houses. This kept us awake and I am sure warned the thief to be wary and avoid this beat. I grew fond of him, and he would see me for the minor illnesses he was prone to.

143

Once I asked him, "Dilbahadur, why do you make this noise? It ruins our sleep."

For this Dilbahadur said, "*Saab*, how else does the robber know I am around?"

This kind of Gurkha logic was tough to beat. As there was no point in arguing, I requested him to reduce the noise he was making.

As I said, he would see me for his health problems, not always minor.

On one such visits I asked him, "What is the problem this time?"

"Same as last time," he said.

"What same as last time?" I asked.

"Woman problem [He used the Hindi word *aurath*]. Last time you gave an injection, and in one day I got cured," he replied.

That was what one shot of penicillin did in those days.

I told him that this was becoming too much and advised him to get married and avoid this risky life of a bachelor. He grinned and went.

Some months later, he came and said, "*Saab*, I have a wife now," and called out, "Dhrama, come here. This is our doctor *Saab*, do *pranam*."

The shy girl did so by touching my feet. I gave her a small gift of ten rupees [a big amount in those days].

While going, he said that now he has a family to manage, and hence he was hiking his nightbeat fee!

After some months, a crestfallen Bahadur came to the clinic. I asked him what had happened.

He said, "Wife ran away."

"Where?" I asked him.

"Village," he replied.

This was news to me, so I asked him "Why?"

"She did not like my night duty, wanted me to change job." Bahadur said.

Sound logic, I thought. Which newly married woman wants her man to be away doing night duty?

I asked him, "What are you going to do?"

"I will go and get her back," he said and asked for some money.

A couple of months later, he came and met with me. He looked happy. He had his wife with him.

I told him, "Hope this time she will stay."

He said, "*Saab*, my hope too is that *this one* will stay."

This one meant another woman. To my eyes, one Nepali woman looked like another.

I asked what had happened to Dhrama. He said he couldn't find her; instead, he found this one.

Quite an enterprising guy, our Dilbahadur!

The second wife stayed put. Produced two sons. Now a grandfather, Dilbahadur visits me once in a while and makes fond enquiries. The attractive grin has never left him all these fifty-odd years.

❖❖◆❖

A Forgetful Affair

I see older people coming to me with complaints of forgetfulness. This is often associated with the onset of dementia, not uncommon in the elderly.

But when Savitha and Deepak Jain came to see me, and Savitha requested in Hindi, "Doctor, please do something, prescribe some medicine for this husband of mine; it is becoming impossible to live with him," I knew something serious had happened between them.

Savitha and Deepak have been my patients for some years now. Well brought up and belonging to an upper-crust Marwari family, they have made Bangalore their home.

I asked her, "What happened to make you so upset?"

"You better ask him why," she replied.

Now it was his turn, "Doctor, yesterday evening we went to Jayanagar market to do our weekly shopping on my scooter. We went to the vegetable and fruit shop first and then as she wanted to buy some flowers, we went there. Afterwards, we went to the bookshop close by, and I drove back home."

He continued, "As the gate was closed, I asked Savitha to open it, but there was no reply, and I found Savitha was not on the pillion. I had not realised she was not riding pillion. I was very worried, and I drove back all the way to Jayanagar and asked the fruit vendor, whether he had seen my wife. For him it was a joke, 'Many women come here; how do I know which one is your wife?' he said. I had no luck in other places either. So, I drove back home only to see Savitha sitting on the steps, of course very angry."

This was becoming interesting.

I asked for her version. "Doctor, he left me at the florist and went to the bookshop. When I went there, he was not to be seen. He had gone home leaving me there. And he did not

146

even know that I was not riding on the pillion. I took an autorickshaw and came home with the bags. Here I found the door locked, and he had the key. I had to wait for an hour for this great man to arrive."

I tried to allay her fears. "But doctor, this is not the first time he has forgotten like this. A month back he had left me high and dry after lunch at a wedding and had gone to the office; he only realised when he came home in the evening. Now you tell me, how am I going to manage my life with him?"

I spent another fifteen minutes trying to reassure her. All the time Deepak was sitting crestfallen. In the end, he said he would make sure such incidents do not happen again. It took some convincing to make them understand that there is no medicine to cure forgetfulness.

This incident happened in the pre-mobile phone days. In the eighties it took only fifteen minutes to commute from Indiranagar to Jayanagar, compared to an hour or more it takes now. If the couple had mobile phones, this kind of mishap would not have happened. One of the many benefits of smartphones is that they help to keep couples within reach of each other.

❖❖◆❖

Philomena and her Adventures

Father D'Souza was the only son of his parents. He had five sisters of whom only one is alive now. He spent part of his life here in the city, and he was the parish priest for the area where I practised. He lived with his old mother. Two of his sisters lived not far from where he lived. They were all my patients.

Father was a sincere person and had a personality to go with his good manners. In his priest's robes, a goatee beard, and a plethoric, bespectacled face, he was very impressive.

147

His eldest sister Elvera was then working in Mumbai and had a property close to where I lived and the other sister, Elizabeth, and her family also lived close by, after their return from the Gulf. Father D' Souza lived most of the time in the church premises in the Cox Town [now called Sarvagnanagar] area but spent the weekends and some evenings in the house belonging to his sister Elvera.

On occasional weekends, I would spend some time with him and his brother-in-law, Robert who also had the same surname, D'Souza.

Philomena was the cook and housekeeper and was with Father D'Souza for a long time and both had roots in the small town of Kapu in the coastal district of South Canara [Karnataka]. Once, she had a severe attack of giddiness and was brought to my clinic. She had no other complaints except for giddiness, which she said she had for some years and that it came and went; she had not gone to any doctor.

I examined her, and while taking her blood pressure, I smelt alcohol.

Could she be *drinking*? I asked her.

At first, she denied it. But later agreed that she did drink from Father's bottle and replaced the exact quantity with water so that the level remained the same!

She pleaded with me not to tell the Father and spoil the good relationship. She also promised me not to touch his bottle. I felt that she would keep the promise of not stealing but was not sure of her quitting the habit. Her dizzy spells were due to very high blood pressure, possibly exacerbated by a strong dose of whisky. I put her on blood pressure medication and, after taking her promise of abstinence, let her go.

Occasionally, I shared a drink with Father and his brother-in-law. On one occasion Father had complained that the whisky sold in the market did not taste as good as it was in the earlier days.

Now I knew *why* Father's whisky did not taste good.

I didn't check with Father about the taste of his whisky after Philomena's promise. Since he didn't complain, I suppose he noticed some improvement in the standards but didn't think to share this with me.

Did Philomena give up drinking?

Father passed away some years later due to heart failure, which he was suffering from for a long time. The staff dispersed, and I did not know where Philomena went until I made a house call to Mr. Benjamin's house. This Benjamin was another Gulf returnee and lived in the same locality. The house call was to see his ailing wife who was not able to come to the clinic. After the house call, as I was about to leave, Benjamin wanted me to have a cup of tea with him.

Now, who do you think brought the tea?

You guessed it right: *Our Philomena!*

Did she smell of alcohol? *Of course, she did.*

I felt it prudent not to reveal her secret to the present employer and make her lose a job and Mr. Benjamin a competent cook.

Matters stood that way when one day Mr. Benjamin brought Philomena to see me as she was having dizzy spells. The earlier scenario was repeated. Philomena had stopped taking her blood pressure pills but had not stopped her alcohol habit.

This time I had to tell her boss about her blood pressure and her alcohol habit. Of course, I did not reveal her habit of stealing. Mr. Benjamin knew about her drinking but said that it was manageable and wanted me to advise her to give up, given her health.

I did my duty. Philomena lived for several years and worked for the Benjamin family till her death due to a stroke. Was her blood pressure under control, and did she give up her alcohol habit? I am not sure as I did not see her in later years.

❖❖◆❖

Paad Pooja: Sole-Searching

In the vernacular heavily influenced by Sanskrit, *paad pooja* translates to feet worship. *Paad* means feet, and *pooja* means worship. We Indians, especially Hindus, see the presence of the divine in everything around us and worship trees, the sun, rain, birds, animals, idols, and going by the newspaper reports even cinema stars!

So, worshipping feet should be no surprise to those who know our ways. Still, one is at liberty to wonder whose feet we are worshipping.

It is a common custom to show respect to our elders, close friends, relatives, those who know more than we do, and those who are in power [e.g., politicians] by folding our hands. In extreme cases, this respect takes the form of bending low and touching the feet. Occasionally, it goes even further, when the person showing respect falls flat on the ground and touches or holds the feet of the recipient of the respect [Temple deities, Swamijis, and Gurujis fall into this category].

I routinely touch the feet of my patients. This is part of my standard examination procedure. I look at the colour and texture, feel the pulses, and check for the presence or absence of infection and sensations. I get a wealth of information from this close inspection. Sometimes I spend more time looking at their feet than at their faces.

Many of my patients, often those whom I see for the first time, are uncomfortable and feel that I, being more educated

150

and informed [according to them], should not be touching their feet. They show their discomfort by a quick withdrawal of their feet away from my probing hands. I have, on occasion, had to use gentle force to keep their feet still.

One elderly gentleman had tears in his eyes and expressed that what I did was wrong. The conversation went as follows:

"Doctor, you should not be touching my feet."

I asked, "Why not?"

"It is wrong, that is why," he said.

"Don't you visit temples?" I asked him.

He said yes, he did.

"Don't you bend down and touch the feet of the deity?"

He said yes, when permitted.

This established, I asked him, "Don't you give me my fee before you go?"

He said yes, and I could see some confusion on his face.

Then I explained to him all the information I obtain when I examine his feet.

So, by touching his feet, I said, "I gain knowledge and also money. In a way, it is better than going to a temple and worshipping a deity and not being sure of receiving what you desire."

He was quiet for a while, and the truth of what I said finally sank in. But the tears kept flowing.

❖❖◆❖

The Case of the Shouting Sardar

It was not a busy day. After the patient's consultation was over, he lingered for a chat, finding no patients waiting. I don't remember what *earthshaking matter* we were discussing, but I do remember the panic knocks on the closed door. This put an end to our gossip, and on opening the door, I found this greatly agitated man.

I asked him, "What is the big hurry? Couldn't you have waited a few more minutes?"

To this, he replied, "Sir, the matter is very urgent. My boss is very sick. He cannot come here; he is in bed and wants you to see him. Please come with me."

He also introduced himself as Ranganathan and that he works for Shardul Singh Majithia, who was overseeing a major hotel building project. I agreed to see this Shardul Singh who seemed to instil a kind of fearful reverence in the underlings, as seen in Ranganathan.

I asked him, "What is your boss's problem?"

For this, he said he did not know and only knew that his boss had not gotten up from bed since morning, was shouting at his staff, and in a bad mood.

Curious, I asked him, "Is he always like this?"

"No sir, he is a very good man; please let us go."

I asked him, "Where is the house?"

He said it was close by and then shared the house's location and street. It was a fifteen-minute walk, and I told Ranganathan that we would walk.

He said, "Doctor, my boss has told me to bring you in his car." He showed me the parked car and I had no option but to agree.

Within ten minutes, we reached the house where the patient resided. No sooner had the car reached the residence than a security guard came running to open the car door and stood aside reverentially. A bit embarrassing was this kind of reception to me, who went about visiting on a second-hand scooter.

At the entrance, another gentleman who introduced himself as Chethan Shetty, took over from Ranganathan and led me inside.

Regarding his unwell boss, he told me this: "Doctor, our boss heads the construction of a hotel chain and he travels a lot. He is in Bangalore to supervise the finish of this star hotel [the present Oberoi on MG road]. He has been here for some months, and once the building is finished and handed over, he will leave this city and will go back to Delhi, where the hotel chain's head office is."

I asked him his boss's name. He said, "Shardul Singh Majithia."

He made me sit in the waiting area and went inside a room to find out if his ill boss would be in a fit condition to see me. As soon as he went inside, I heard loud shouting but could not make out what the shouting was all about. Shetty came out wiping his forehead with a handkerchief and said, "Boss is angry because I have not offered you tea!"

I asked him, "Can I go in?"

He said, "Please have a cup of tea and then go; if not he will again shout at me."

I told him not to worry; I would manage his boss and, without waiting for Shetty's reply, I went in.

What did I see?

A room with all the windows closed and, on the floor, next to the bed, lay Mr. Shardul Singh. A woman was massaging his feet with some oil.

At my sight, Shardul Singh lifted his head and said, "Doctor *Saab*, please take a seat," and directed me to a chair. I made my way there and sat.

Now Shardul Singh said loudly to that woman, "Wipe out all the oil and get the hell out from here. Come again same time tomorrow morning." The masseuse did what was told and hurriedly left.

"Doctor, I am very grateful for you having come to see me. I have to rely on these inefficient people to get work done. See this house, it is nearly a month since I have been residing here, and I am fed up trying to get work done." All this was told in *finely accented British English*.

Somehow this huge Sardar with an unkempt beard, with a cap on, and most of the body bare except for a pair of ill-fitting shorts, didn't go with that kind of accent.

To get him back to the point, I asked him, "What is the problem? Why have you called me? You do not look all that sick."

He said, "Doc, you don't know my misery. Every time I visit this city, I go down with some problem or the other. Last time it was diarrhoea which nearly killed me. This time it is my breathing problem. My nose is blocked, and I have to breathe through my mouth. The whole night I was awake because of this."

I knew his problem: severe nasal allergy. But before I discussed this problem, I was curious to know why he was getting his feet massaged. I asked him.

He said, "Doctor, my late mother used this method to cure coughs and colds. It has worked for me, but this time it has not worked though I am getting this done for a few days."

I couldn't help but laugh. This UK-educated Sardar remained a *rustic* at heart.

As I mentioned earlier, ragweed's proliferation contributed to widespread respiratory issues in those years, in the undeveloped and swampy lands that would become Indiranagar and HAL 1st and 2nd stages and our Sardar was a victim of this. He fortunately had no asthma but was having severe nasal allergy. I explained this to him.

He said, "I need to be here for another two weeks. I have lots of work and I cannot depend on these Ranga and Shetty types to do this. I need to be fit and up and about. Please do something urgent and see that I can breathe and sleep at night and be active during the day."

Symptomatic treatment for nasal allergy is easy. I prescribed some nasal drops and a course of oral steroids plus antihistamines and asked him to report back after a few days.

I was getting ready to go but he would have none of it. He let out a shout, "*Oyae, Shattttyy!*"

Poor Shetty came running. "Can't you see that doctor is going? Get us some tea."

Shetty said, "Sir, I will get it," and disappeared from the scene before Sardar abused him more.

I couldn't help asking him, "Mr. Singh, why do you need to shout at him to get this small job done?"

He said, "You don't know doctor, my job is to build hotels, and I have to deal with local people. Across the world it is the same, I have found out that the louder the command, better the result."

Though I did not agree with this surmise, I thought it best to be quiet.

Cups of tea arrived. Sardar told the standing Shetty to also have a cup and then take me back to my clinic.

He asked me for my visiting fees. I told him and he said he would send it later.

On the way back, Shetty told me about his boss. "I have worked with a lot of people in this construction business, and I am yet to come across a more decent person than Shardul Singh Sir."

That evening, a pack of sweets and an envelope arrived containing five hundred-rupee notes—a *princely amount* in those days.

❖❖◆❖❖

Dr. John and his Many Illnesses

When I first met Dr. Jacob John, he was seventy-five and I was thirty-five. For the next fifteen years, until he passed away at ninety, he remained my patient and friend. He worked in the railways and had retired some twenty-odd years ago. And had forgotten most of the medicine which he was then familiar with and was virtually a layperson as far as medical knowledge went. In fact, what little remained of that knowledge interfered with the diagnosis and treatment when he took ill, real or imaginary.

It took me a while before I realised Dr. John was a hypochondriac and had a very fertile imagination and that he highly exaggerated his symptoms. He was living close to my branch office, along with his aged wife Sosamma. This was within walking distance and commuting was not an issue for him. Often, I would find him waiting for me and he would pour out his complaints.

When I first saw him complaining of severe pain in the belly, I made him lie down on the examination couch and did a detailed check. All sorts of serious possible causes went through my mind which included volvulus, ulcer disease and the like. Except for a mildly enlarged liver which I attributed to visceroptosis [descent of organs due to ageing], I found nothing wrong. Even while I was examining him, he started feeling better, and I gave him a prescription for an antispasmodic tablet [which he came to call *yellow pill*]. Later, I realised he would have gotten better, whatever I gave him.

Dr. John was one of the fittest elderly people I have seen—medium built, well-muscled [weightlifter in his younger days], low blood pressure and pulse, and excellent digestion. One could not have asked for better health. But Dr. John did not believe so and did not like it when I told him so.

I soon realised that he wanted to spend time visiting me and talking. He either found or *made* many opportunities for this. He had four sons, fifteen grandchildren, and many great-grandchildren whose numbers and names he could not recollect. Someone or the other would not be well and it was a handy reason for him to visit me.

He would come with a problem and start as, "Doctor, you know my third son Suresh, his son…." He would sit there trying to recall that grandson's name, failing which he would curse his poor memory, and proceed that the grandson was unwell, and the Mumbai doctor had prescribed some medicine. He would take out a chit, tell me the name, and ask, "Is this the correct medicine? I have not heard of this medicine."

Of course, he had not. When he was in service, this drug was not available. Even if it was, he would not have remembered. I told him that it was a good drug. This seemed to mollify him a bit.

While reluctantly taking leave he said, "You doctors give very strong medicines, not good for health." I kept quiet as there was an element of truth in what he said, though I did not like him including me in that group.

Another time he came after visiting the chemist. He said, "The present-day chemists are not well-trained. I asked for Novopone tablet, and he said there is no such medicine."

"Of course, it is not there anymore," I told him.

But he was not convinced. "Such a good medicine and he does not have it. OK, you give me something for my gas," he said.

There was one real problem, however, which in addition to causing him trouble also gave him a valid excuse to see me. For a man of his age, Dr. John's blood pressure was very low. Unlike other elderly, his BP never went up. It remained the same from his teenage years to his present ripe old age.

While it did not trouble him when he was young, now it did and caused occasional dizzy spells. Any and every head-related complaint like headache, buzzing, loss of balance, and slow walking, were all attributed to this low pressure, and times without number he would visit my clinic to get his blood pressure checked. He knew when I would be having a rush of patients and when I would be free.

Once his wife came and asked me, "Doctor, will you please come and see my husband? He is not getting up, and says he feels like vomiting. I tried giving him *Kashayam* [a kind of home remedy], but he insists on seeing you."

Of course, the poor lady had no choice, and neither did I. So, I walked up to his house. I saw Dr. lying comfortably. Did I hear a small snore? Maybe.

Sosamma rudely woke him, "*Enda* [hello] doctor is here."

He abruptly sat up and had a real attack of vertigo. He shouted, "*Ayyo!*" and fell back on the bed.

Sosamma ran to get some hot water though I did not know what for. She said that whenever this happened, he would drink a cup of hot water and become better.

Sudden sitting up and turning his head had made his blood pressure drop and kinked his neck arteries, producing a momentary compromise to his blood supply to the brain. It got corrected soon after he lay down. I sat beside him and took the BP, which was normal [to him], made him slowly get up, stand, and had him sit on a chair.

His giddiness had gone! He was full of praise not for my knowledge but for my *Kaiguna* [a word in Kannada which meant, just you being there near me or some such medically non-attributable quality].

This mildly forgetful [onset of dementia], hypochondriac Dr. John developed one of those belly aches of his. This happened when I was on leave. As I was not able to see him, I asked him to see Dr. Shankar who also practised close by and looked after my patients when I was not available.

Dr. John told his wife, "That boy is never available when I need him. He now wants me to see this strange doctor, I don't want to go there, I will wait for him to get back."

"But he will not be back for the next four days," said Sosamma.

"Last time he gave me this yellow pill, I will take it and wait till evening. If not better, I will go and see this doctor," he replied.

By evening, though better, he was not fully relieved of his pain. They went to see Dr. Shankar. Dr. John described his belly ache in *graphic* detail. Like I did when I first saw him with this type of complaint some years back, Dr. Shankar too made him lie down and examined him. He found Dr. John's liver to be enlarged. Having not found anything wrong, but worried about the liver, he advised a specialist consultation in a hospital.

In those days no scanning facility was available and enlarged liver in the elderly who had repeated episodes of pain sometimes necessitated a liver biopsy.

Much against his wishes, he was admitted, and tests were done, which included swallowing liquid barium and taking serial X-rays of the belly. Dr. John stayed for three days in the hospital. By the second day, his belly pain disappeared, and all the tests done were normal. He was given a pill that was the same as the one prescribed by me [What Dr. John called the yellow pill]!

A chastened Dr. John met with me and said, "You should not take leave and make me go to a strange doctor. He made me go to the hospital for a liver problem."

"Why did you not tell him that you have had this for ages, and it was not a serious problem [visceroptosis]?" I asked him.

"I told him, but he insisted, as I was having continuous pain, to go to the hospital," he said.

I defended Dr. Shankar and told him, "In a way it is good that all the tests were done, and they are normal."

Dr. John said, "Yes, but the medicine they gave me is the same as you had given without doing all these tests."

"You made me spend a lot of money," he added as an afterthought.

He kept seeing me for one problem or the other and I was able to manage him without any further tests for many years. Our fifteen years of relationship ended with his death at the ripe age of ninety.

Between his wife and me, we managed his slowly progressive dementia quite well.

❖❖◆❖

'The One More Thing' Syndrome

I spend anywhere from fifteen minutes to half an hour, sometimes more, with each patient. Often, when I finish with the process of history taking, examination, and treatment advice and just feel relieved that my brain can now get a few minutes' rest before the next patient comes in, the patient, instead of taking his or her leave, pipes in, "Doc, *one more thing*, I forgot to tell you."

And then proceeds to tell me that 'one more thing'.

This 'one more thing' often turns out to be the most important thing, and it will make me rethink my diagnosis and the treatment I had advised! Also, it means re-examination and spending more time!

Whenever this 'one more thing' comes up, which is not infrequent, I have often felt like throwing my stethoscope at the patient. I have *never* done it, though.

When Mr. Shailesh Gupta saw me, he was well past sixty years old and had been under treatment by several doctors. Lately, I have avoided new patients as it meant taking responsibility and always being available, either in person or on the telephone. However, I am still available to the few remaining old patients, 24/7.

Nonetheless, occasionally, I am forced to see a new patient because of pressure from someone close to me, and this Gupta was one such.

He had a sheaf of old records with him, and by the look of it, he had come prepared for a long consultation. He also had a paper on which he had written down all the questions he meant to ask me. He proceeded to tell me all his complaints one by one which included tiredness, feeling lightheaded, backache, belching and lack of sleep. Most of these vague complaints generally have no lasting solution and one does not find a diagnosis which explains all these complaints.

Going through all his records I found multiple drugs given for his diabetes, borderline high blood pressure, lack of sleep and, to a good measure, there was a prescription for Vitamin D, calcium, and B complex. I counted the number of drugs, and it came to nine of them. Most were to be taken twice a day, and a few three times a day.

I asked him, "Mr. Gupta, how do you manage to keep track of these many drugs?"

"I don't; my wife does," was his reply.

Gupta had found an easy way out. In my mind, I was certain that his wife, however sharp she may be, would miss out on some.

I found that he hardly did any exercise; I spent some time advising him on the importance of diet and regular exercise. I had told him I would only see him again if he agreed to let me reduce his medication. So, despite feeling many of the drugs could be safely stopped, I refrained from doing so during this consultation, which took more than half an hour—twice my usual time.

Gupta sincerely thanked me for the time and was about to leave when he turned around and said, "Doc, one more thing that I forgot to tell you: I have this urge to pass urine frequently, and it is a bother, especially at night."

"Have you told your doctor?" I asked.

"I told him, and he said not to worry; it is because of my diabetes," he replied.

I made him come back and proceeded to take the history of this complaint. I then examined his genitals and groin area, where I found a mild fungal infection. I deduced his symptoms to be due to an enlarged prostate. He needed to do some tests including an ultrasound scan, and after the tests, he needed to see a doctor. This took another fifteen minutes of explanation.

Where should he go after the tests? He requested another consult.

I had to agree.

Thus, Mr. Gupta became another regular patient, all because of this 'one more thing'. He did have an enlarged prostate and needed medication. Over time, I was able to get his drug numbers down to five.

No mean achievement, don't you agree?

✧✧✦✧

The Unlikely Friendship

Kempamma lived in the nearby slum called Marappan Palya. Most residents were poor and worked as labourers and factory workers and some of them were petty traders running small kiosks. Kempamma initially came to me as a patient and later as a sweeper, in and around my clinic premises. This job took just about half an hour. By her good nature and manners, she became close to me.

Needless to say, whenever she and her family fell ill, the treatment was free. She had lost her husband, had one son, and was the sole breadwinner, which she managed by doing odd jobs that included the part-time work she did for me.

As I said, she had one son, and he was Nanjunda.

When I first saw this boy, he must have been ten years old. His mother brought him to me as he had festering sores on the fingers and toes with some on both palms, was undernourished with a gaunt expressionless face, and had a fever. These made him look more miserable than he was. It took anti-scabies [a kind of skin infection] application along with penicillin injections to get him better in the next ten days. During these ten days, he couldn't go to the local school.

163

A month later I had gone on a house call, and outside was Nanjunda washing a car parked in that house. I asked him, "Why are you not in school?"

"The teachers beat me," he said.

"Why so?" I asked.

He kept quiet. When I insisted, he said, "I fight with other boys."

I now knew the answer. He, coming from a poor social background, was easy prey for other children. Taking a promise that he would go back to school, I went into the house to see the patient. After I finished, I asked the patient about the car wash and Nanjunda. The man was all praise for the boy and said he was sincere and did a very good job.

A couple of days later when I asked Kempamma about Nanjunda's school-going, she evaded and told me that he now washed three cars in the morning and one in the evening and was thereby supplementing her income.

Another time she brought him was for diarrhoea. While examining him I smelt tobacco. Suspicious, I asked him about smoking. He said once in a way he did smoke a *beedi* and further added that all his friends did so. I spent some time telling him why he needed to stop smoking. His mother intoned saying it was useless to argue with him, only to get a blistering stare from the son.

His school-going and education stopped after 5th standard, and he would boast that he could read and write Kannada and English and that was enough education for him. His car washing in the morning and evening left him with some spare time which he spent idling with similarly placed youngsters close to where my practice was located.

Once, curious to know what they were doing, I asked him, and he said they played the numbers game. Later I realised it was a type of gambling. Naturally, this pastime led to disputes and fistfights.

Next, he graduated to become a gambling agent. This illegal activity made him come under the eye of the law and he was recognised as a petty criminal. In one of his fights, he was even arrested and later released due to his mother's pleading and his assurance. He continued his activities and his legitimate business of car washing and painting that he had picked up. This and the other unlawful activities got him enough income to lead a fair but risky life.

Shambu, like Nanjunda, was also a school dropout but unlike Nanjunda, Shambu took to honest work. His life began in a hotel as a help in the kitchen and later graduated to become a server. He then branched out and started his small eatery in Marappan Palya where our Nanjunda too plied his trade of car washing and other sundry legal and often illegal activities.

Shambu was much older, married, and had school-going children. His hotel catered to poor and lower middle-class men and women and was very popular.

Nanjunda was a frequent visitor and his reputation as a troublemaker preceded him. He would often walk away without paying. Shambu took it as a part of this business as there were several such freebooters like the beat policeman, the local health-inspector, and the like. As long as Nanjunda alone took his meal/breakfast, Shambu did not mind. But when he started coming with his gang, it became too much and Shambu had to tell Nanjunda to pay and eat. This did not please our hero.

Strange things started happening to the eatery. Shambu's assistant Raja would come early in the morning to tidy up and prepare the items for breakfast. Then other workers would come and the place was ready for service by half past seven in the morning. On one such morning, Raja found a mass of

165

dirt sitting on the steps of the eatery. It took a lot of effort to get rid of the offending, foul-smelling dirt and restore the place. The lingering smell remained till later in the afternoon.

Another day, the autorickshaw that brought supplies to the eatery was stopped and the supplies were looted by a masked gang. Another day some unknown customer raised a hue and cry as he found a dead lizard in the *idly sambar* plate. This made the regular customers wonder about the hygiene of the place.

This was repeated a week later. Gradually the number of customers started to decrease. It took some time for Shambu to realise that Nanjunda was behind this. He went to the police and told them of his suspicion.

By then the police and Nanjunda had become *buddies of sorts*, as he would help the police in some of their cases, kind of an informer, so to speak. They told Shambu to provide proof that Nanjunda was responsible. This was tough. Matters stood like this when someone told Shambu to seek my help.

We from the coast form a kind of fraternity and come to know each other quickly. I knew him both as a patient and as a reasonably successful hard-working hotelier. So, one fine day, a worried-looking Shambu came to see me and told me the story of his misery and his suspicion. I told him that I would do my best but could not promise, as I knew that Nanjunda followed his own counsel and may not heed my advice.

Since Nanjunda started doing well in his activities, legal or otherwise, his mother Kempamma had stopped doing the odd jobs, though she still sought my help whenever she fell ill. I sent word asking her to find time to see me.

One morning, she came to see me and asked why I wanted to see her. Was it for some mischief her son was involved in? This Kempamma was different from the one I was used to.

Though civil in her attitude as before, she spoke with newfound confidence and was well-groomed in an expensive *saree* and blouse with a pair of gold bangles adorning both her wrists. She was looking good.

I complimented her and then proceeded to tell her the story. She kept quiet for a while and then said, rather noncommittally, "I will ask him to see you," and took her leave.

Few days later, our hero dropped in.

"What *Saar*, you wanted to see me?" he asked.

"Didn't your mother tell you?" I asked.

"No, she only told me to see you."

Here I felt Kempamma had played her cards well. Had she told him why, then it was possible he would have avoided seeing me. So, she had just told him to see me and not the reason why.

I then told him about the suffering Shambu was going through and the loss he had to put up with. Nanjunda listened without committing yes or no. His silence told me that he was the perpetrator.

He stood up and before leaving, told me, "Tell that fool that going to the police will not help but will only give him more trouble." He left without promising anything but issued another threat to be conveyed to the hapless hotelier.

What happened next is much more interesting.

Shambu hesitated to bill him; Nanjunda issued a threat, "Do you want dirt on your entrance once again?" His gang too would visit and pay for the food. There was no trouble at all from these "honest citizens".

At the time of writing this story some years back, the truce was not only holding but had become strong, and whenever

Shambu had any trouble with his labour or with the civic authorities or when he needed more labour, he sought help from Nanjunda.

Later one day, when Shambu had come for some health issue, he told me, "*Saar*, Nanjundappa, is a good man at heart."

Nanjunda had graduated and become Nanjundappa, an honourific addition of *appa*, which is like saying, Nanjunda Sir!

❖❖◆❖❖

Magic Cure

Dr. K.S. Hande was a general practitioner and like me had gone through difficult times in the early years of his practice. When patients are few and far between, one has lots of idle time. This time sadly must be spent in the clinic, as one cannot afford to be elsewhere for fear of losing even that occasional patient.

While my pastime was reading, his was to stand outside his clinic and watch the humanity go by. One day, some thirty-five years ago, when he was indulging in this favourite pastime, to his surprise he saw one of his patients who had visited him a few days earlier pass by cheerfully, waving a greeting.

This patient really had no business walking around so cheerfully because when he visited the doctor, he was a very sick person with pneumonia, as confirmed by an X-ray. How then did he get well? Why did he not turn up the next day as advised? Did he go to another doctor and get better? Did I do anything wrong? Was my fee too much that drove this man away from me? These were the worrisome thoughts that Dr. Hande had.

He got the patient to come in and asked him, "What had happened? Why did you not turn up the next day?"

"What *Saar* [Sir], you gave *magic* injection that day; the next day my fever went, the second day my cough went, and yesterday I ate well and felt fit, and now I am on my way to work. I did not come because your one injection of that *magic* medicine cured me," the patient said.

A quick examination revealed complete clearance of his lungs!

Dr. Hande had given the patient 400,000 units of procaine penicillin. That was how the drug acted in those days!

One cannot think of such cures *now*.

We have today made a mess of the treatment of infections by indiscriminate use of antibiotics and the germs have developed resistance to most antibiotics, and society is paying a heavy price for the physician's folly!

A dreaded time may soon arrive when we see patients dying due to these multidrug-resistant infections.

❖❖◆❖❖

What is Success?

Babanna [his real name is Anil Menon] was a bright student and highly inquisitive by nature. Once I had asked him what he wanted to become in life. He told me that he wanted to become the chief of a big company, like Bill Gates. He did his college and his Engineering, all with flying colours. I thought he would head for the United States and pursue his dream of becoming Bill Gates.

For a few years, I did not hear from him, and his mother, when asked, said that her son has not gone to the United States and was working for a local company. She also told me that Babanna was reluctant to see me, as he was afraid that I would scold him. She did not appear to be very happy with his progress.

169

I told her, "I will not do such a thing," and asked her to get him to see me.

Babanna came to see me. He had changed. The last I saw him was some three to four years before. A clean-shaven Babanna was now sporting a goatee beard and had put on weight.

I asked him as an opening gambit, "Babanna, what are you doing these days?"

He said, "Nothing, just whiling away time."

"What happened to the job?" I asked.

"I quit," he said.

All this was news to me. Here was a bright young man, with the ambition of becoming another Bill Gates, jobless and rootless.

I asked him, "Why?"

He said, "I cannot get along with people. I find everyone selfish and money-minded. I do not fit in with any job environment. I have changed jobs three times in the past three years."

I asked him questions to find out if I was dealing with some mental health problems like depression. He was in perfect mental health, and his ideals were such that he would find it tough to get on with most people.

I asked him what he wanted to do.

"I am planning to do something on my own which is less stressful," he replied.

I wished him the best of luck. He bid goodbye and left.

After his parents moved to a different part of the city, I lost track of the family until a few days ago, when Babanna came to see me with a young woman. They had come to invite me to their wedding.

While congratulating them, I asked him, "What are you now doing?"

He said, "I am running a stationary store, and my soon-to-be wife teaches in a school."

Both appeared very happy. Our future Bill Gates is now a happy shop owner and has no regrets about being one.

Another story that shows that success and happiness are *relative* terms.

❖❖◆❖

5

WHEN FAITH GETS FUNNY

A Puzzled Pharmacist

At 7 pm one evening many years ago, I received a panic-stricken call from a nearby chemist. He said some of my patients were creating a ruckus in front of his shop. I asked him why. He said, "Sir, the medicine you prescribed is not available, and they don't believe me. They are shouting at me that you told them it was available."

I wanted to know the name of the patient causing this trouble. He returned after ascertaining the name and said the chief troublemaker's name was Kishenchand.

This Kishenchand was part of a group of carpenters from Rajasthan who had made Bangalore their home. The building boom here had attracted all sorts of artisans, and being very hard-working, they were assured of regular work. They are a hardy and simple lot with ready, contented smiles and were usually docile but volatile when provoked [as evidenced by the frequent brawls amongst them on weekends].

For them, I am the last word in medicine, I am a *mister cure-all*, and there was no disease on earth that I couldn't cure. This kind of blind faith is quite frightening, to say the least. Often, I have tried telling them facts to the contrary, only to be told that I am being too modest!

Living in groups, often on the construction sites, and eating and drinking by the wayside, they are very prone to illnesses, and Kishenchand had come that morning with a fever of three days' duration. I remember prescribing some paracetamol [acetaminophen] tablets. As was his habit, he had asked me before leaving with the prescription, "*Saab* [sir], I hope this is easily available." I had guaranteed that it was easily available.

Now here was a chemist claiming this common drug was not available. So, I asked him, "How come you don't stock paracetamol?"

He said, "Sir, the medicine you have prescribed is *PUO – three days*. We don't have this drug. I have even searched the drug directory, and it is not mentioned even in that."

I told him to dispense paracetamol and to tell Kishenchand to see me later with the medication. After getting their medicine, the group left without causing any physical harm to the chemist.

PUO is the short form for pyrexia of unknown origin or [I don't know what is causing this fever]. Normally, that is what I write in my notes. What must have happened is that instead of writing this in the case notes, I had written it on the prescription for the chemist.

The Hindi-speaking simple Rajasthani, who thinks his doctor is one who commits no error, and the chemist, who was puzzled at the strange name, were thus at loggerheads.

When I tried explaining to the simple carpenter what had transpired, he still would not blame me but kept saying that the chemist was insolent and that he should have checked with me first instead of saying that the drug was not available and getting into a needless argument with him and his friends.

I kept quiet.

❖❖◆❖

174

White Coat Hypertension

Many illnesses are directly linked to brain activity. This is illustrated by the case of a patient who presented herself recently.

This patient, who is on medication for high blood pressure, records her pressure at home, and often it is within the normal range. But whenever I take her pressure, it is way above the normal. I tried reassuring her that this is a well-known phenomenon, and explained to her that we have even coined the term "white coat hypertension" for this.

She was not convinced and said, "I am a calm person. I have known you for many years, and there is nothing here to get excited about [this is true, especially given my age!]. Your measuring instrument is showing the wrong reading."

I have learnt not to argue with some patients, and this is one of them. I said, "Right then, you bring your instrument tomorrow, and we will check the pressure with both the machines and see which one shows the correct reading."

She came the next day. I don't know *which one* of us was more anxious! She took her blood pressure with her instrument, which showed an even higher reading than the one from the previous day! Then I took her pressure, using her instrument first and then mine. The readings were lower than hers!

She was now convinced but wanted to know why my reading was lower than hers.

"The excitement was *already over* when I took the reading; therefore, the figures were lower," I said, half in jest.

I presume she will have more faith in me and my equipment henceforth!

❖❖◆❖

175

Astrologer Approved Appendectomy

During the last fifty-odd years of family medical practice, I have encountered many beliefs, which most of us will find odd. But to those who believe, these are literally life-and-death matters.

Ramaswamy is a believer in certain auspicious and inauspicious hours during the day. He will refrain from all activities during these inauspicious hours and stays put in the house. He is certain that he will meet with an accident if he goes out of the house, and any decision taken then will only end in disaster.

To help him decide which are the auspicious hours and which are not, there are ready-to-help almanacs, prepared by erudite pundits. Ramaswamy regularly refers to these to decide if the time is right or not. This applies to seeing his doctor [me] also.

Once it so happened that he developed severe pain in the abdomen and his wife Shamala called me and requested me to come and see him at home. Within five minutes of her call, Ramaswamy called to tell me to come after an hour, as only then this *rahukalam* [inauspicious hour] gets over.

I asked him, "What about your pain?"

"I will manage," he replied.

So, I went to his home at the appointed time and found him in bed with a hot water bag on his belly. It was obvious that he was in severe pain. It did not take long for me to diagnose an acute attack of appendicitis which needed urgent surgery. I explained the situation and the urgency.

Ramaswamy was not worried about the impending surgery, but his worry was about the right time. He asked his wife to get the almanac. After spending some time referring to it and calculating, he told me, "I will get it done tomorrow afternoon, that is the right time."

This put me in a quandary. An appendix does not wait for *his right time* to burst and cause severe complications. I told him so.

He said, "If I get operated on before that time, the operation will kill me."

We had no option but he agreed to get admitted as it was not 'rahukalam'. I got in touch with the surgeon and the hospital and organised his admission. I discussed the problem with the surgeon. The surgeon had an easy solution. He said, "I will sedate him, and he will not know whether it is a good time or a bad time. It is important that we do the surgery immediately and avoid complications."

Ramaswamy needed painkillers and after some preliminary tests, he was operated upon the next morning, and he made an uneventful recovery.

He came to know that the surgery was done in 'rahukalam' by accident. He was going through the discharge summary and found the details of the procedure and the timings.

Until then he was normal. Two weeks after discharge, he began developing vague pains in his belly and back and the surgeon and I were helpless in making him believe that these were not due to the surgery. He kept blaming me for the problems he was then having.

Fortunately, he stuck with me, and in the course of time, these psychological complaints receded. He never missed an opportunity to remind me about the big risk I had taken in treating him, claiming that while it resolved his other issues, it triggered a host of new complaints.

❖❖◆❖

A Love Story, *Rahukalam*-Style

Swaminathan must have been in his early fifties when this story transpired. As it happens with us general practitioners, most patients [who are our regulars] and their families often get close to us and use us as intermediaries to settle problems unrelated to health. Quite a few of these are due to flawed interpersonal relationships, and an unbiased family friend's advice comes in handy and is acceptable to all the parties concerned.

Swamy, as I came to call him, is another staunch believer in this *rahukalam* business. Retired from a successful corporate life, he had chosen to settle in my area of practice and became a sort of friend over the years. His son was married and was well-settled in Mumbai [then Bombay]. His only problem [from his angle] was his daughter Nirmala. She was a good-looking woman of thirty-odd years when this incident happened.

He once told me that my practice would greatly improve if I changed my morning clinic hours from 8.30 am to 8 am as 8.30 am was inauspicious and he was worried that starting work at this time, day in and day out, was not good. I did not heed his advice. That I continued to do reasonably well did not deter him from his belief in 'rahukalam'.

Nirmala, after she finished her graduation, much against the wishes of her parents, decided to do her postgraduate studies and trained as a schoolteacher. She was very happy being a schoolteacher and thoroughly enjoyed her job.

Though she was happy, her parents were not. One reason was that the teachers' job was not in keeping with their standards and the other was that she was unwilling to get married, and they wanted me to have a word with her regarding these two matters.

178

As my telling them that a schoolteacher's job was very satisfying fell on deaf years, I said, I would talk to her, more to satisfy them and not really to dissuade the girl from her job or unwillingness to marry.

One forenoon Nirmala came to see me and said, "What is it, Doctor? You wanted to see me? Dad told me. Is there any problem with him?"

I said, "There is no problem with him, just that he is worried about you not getting married and he thinks you are not interested."

For this she said, "Doctor, it is not that I am not interested, but they want it the traditional way—the whole lot of them coming to interview me and this *matching of horoscopes'* business. I would rather remain unmarried than go through this humiliating process."

I had to agree and told her that I would tell her father to try and change the interview process when the next proposal arrived.

The next prospective match duly arrived, and, surprisingly for Iyer Brahmins, the other party agreed that the boy and girl would meet separately, followed by a meeting of the parents. This was duly agreed upon. A time and venue were fixed for the meeting between Nirmala and the boy [unless he is married, the man remains a boy!].

Nirmala and Ramkrishna met, and it was a sort of love at first sight. Nirmala came home and told the good news to her father, post lunch.

Swamy should have been very happy, but he was instead very unhappy. He told Nirmala, "You were supposed to meet him this evening; how come you met with him in the morning? You should have asked me. You met with him and spent time in 'rahukalam', a very bad time!"

Nirmala would have none of this belief of her father's. She told him in no uncertain terms to go ahead and fix a date as early as possible for her wedding. For every problem there is a solution. The family priest suggested some propitiatory ceremony to counter this meeting at the inauspicious time, and the marriage eventually took place.

Swamy expected some problems and continues to harbour worries. Nirmala and Ramkrishna went to Australia and have been there for several years. Nirmala continues her job as a schoolteacher. The place they live is much hotter than Bangalore, and my friend Swamy and his wife visit there every year.

Once after his return, Swamy told me, "You know, Doctor, they are in that damn place; it is boiling hot. It is all due to their first meeting in 'rahukalam'!"

✦✦✦✦

The House That Ate a Compass

Narayanappa was a successful building construction contractor and real estate dealer. Even when this story was written, Bangalore was showing the signs of a real estate boom and Narayanappa was one of the early beneficiaries. He and his family have been my patients for some years and as it happens in any family which has growing up children, there were frequent visits to me for one illness or the other. Narayanappa himself was a healthy, well-built man though slightly overweight.

Lately however, the family's visits had become rare, which I had attributed to his children growing up and his moving to another part of the locality where there were a couple of doctors practising and naturally, I thought that he had shifted loyalties and was seeking help from them.

So, when the call for a house visit came from him, I was a bit surprised. At the other end, it was Narayanappa himself talking. He said, "It has been two years since I have seen you because we have been healthy and there was no need to visit, but now there is serious sickness with my wife. She has a high fever and is not even able to get up from the bed. Will you please come and see her here?"

I had been to his housewarming ceremony, and the location was familiar because other patients of mine also lived in that area. After the morning session was over, I drove to his house. Try as I might, I couldn't locate his house. I was sure I was in the correct neighbourhood and on the correct street.

There was a petty grocery shop in the same street, and it was still there. I went and asked the shopkeeper as to the location of Mr. Narayanappa's house. He gave precise directions and said, "That house which has its back facing the street and the front facing the back of the house on the next street—you will not miss it, *even if you try.*"

This house was easy enough to find. It was in the same location as it was a few years back but looked very different. While all the houses had their front facing the road, this one had the windows of the rear of the house facing the street!

Despite the shopkeepers' directions, I still had some misgivings about this being Narayanappa's house. Hesitantly, I opened the small gate leading to a narrow passage, and next to the gate was a small board that said that the main door was at the back.

So, that's how it was. The main entry was from the back of the house. Now I could make out the extensive modification the house had undergone to create this *monstrosity* [to my eyes]. The house appeared as though it had been turned around in a kind of semicircle.

I rang the bell and Narayanappa welcomed me and took me inside.

181

Examination and prescription writing did not take much time, and I could now ask him about the house's transformation, or [*malformation*].

He said, "I came to know Mr. S, an expert in *Vasthu* architecture, and met some friends who had built their houses following Vasthu principles. They have done very well in their lives. Before I made these changes to the house, I was not doing all that well and as you know the family was not doing well health-wise, and we used to visit you very often. Since I made these alterations, we hardly have had any sickness, and I have done very well in my business."

I could very well believe this, though I had my doubts about how this had happened. I refrained from saying so. The house looked ghastly from inside and outside, but he seemed to be happy.

I saw a new Maruti car outside. In those days, this wonder car had just entered the market and had a three-year wait period, and Narayanappa owned one! Was Vasthu working *here also*?

I asked him about it. He said, "Maybe, but I bought it after paying a 20,000 rupees premium from someone who had it allotted." Even after paying this added sum, he felt that Vasthu had helped him to become the proud owner of this much sought-after car.

Later, I came to know that this belief in the direction of the house [most preferred direction is that the entry door and the water source face the east], is not uncommon and is widespread even in other eastern countries like China, Thailand, and Japan; it is popularly called *Feng Shui*.

My architect friend told me that house builders are increasingly becoming Vasthu-conscious and are requesting architects to design their homes keeping in mind the principles of Vasthu.

It has done Narayanappa and his family good; who am I to question how this has come about?

❖❖◆❖

To Lie, or Not to Lie?

When I first met Venkataramanappa, it was when I went to see his grandson who was unwell. You may wonder how we doctors of yesteryear made so many house calls which the doctors of today do not. There are many reasons. But the main reason is a great improvement in transportation now. Those days, hardly anyone possessed a car, and getting a very sick person to the doctor was difficult.

Getting the doctor to the patient was an easier option, and we doctors too did not mind. Commuting was easy, and the city roads were less congested to negotiate, especially in the layouts located on the periphery of the city. There were very few hospitals where one could go directly and the ones that did exist were far away and not easy to access.

I went to his house one evening and rang the bell. The lady of the house, Subhadra opened the door and led me inside. I had to pass through the living room to go to the room where the sick boy was lying.

I found the old man sitting cross-legged on a settee with a towel spread on his folded legs, and he was gently and rhythmically, clapping his hands. It appeared as though he was silently praying. I asked Subhadra, his daughter-in-law, "What is he doing?"

She said, "Doctor, it is his way of swatting mosquitoes. See the dead mosquitoes on the towel spread below."

I saw; the towel was black with dead mosquitoes. Not for nothing was our locality then called *Mosquito Nagar!* The present residents cannot imagine what a swampy, unhealthy place this was forty years back. After checking the boy, writing a prescription, and drinking the customary cup of tea, I left the place.

Venkataramanappa's family was a pious and orthodox Brahmin family, steeped in tradition and rituals. His son

183

worked in the state secretariat, as a middle-level officer and was one of the non-corrupt officials, and the family managed with his salary and the old man's pension.

Ten years passed and when he was about eighty, Venkataramanappa suffered a stroke. Unlike these days, we then managed stroke patients at home. He was conscious but unable to swallow. Feeding was done by a feeding tube and urine was drained by a catheter. The daughter-in-law and son were taught how to keep him clean so that he would not get bedsores. Despite all this attention, a bedridden patient's days are numbered, which is true even today with all the advances.

So, it proved in Venkataramanappa's case. One forenoon, when I was busy in the clinic, Sudhakar, the grandson came running and asked me to hurry over to see his granddad, who had stopped moving. When I asked him about breathing, the youngster said he had not observed.

The house was a few kilometres away. Telling the waiting patients about the seriousness of the case and requesting them to wait, I took my bag and rushed to the patient's home.

Anxious son and daughter-in-law were waiting.

Before I went to the room where the patient lay, the daughter-in-law called me aside and asked, "Doctor, in case he is very serious and the end is near, will you let us know? We need to shift him to the front room. If he breathes his last in this room, it will be a problem for all of us. We will not be able to use the front entrance and must go all around the house to enter and you know how difficult it is if we need to do this for the next thirteen days".

I could see her reason and her common-sense approach. I went inside to have a look at the patient. He was dead. I made a show of examination and told the daughter-in-law and son, "He is barely alive; we will shift him to the other room."

184

I helped them to lift the body to the appropriate room [*Vasthu*-wise] and again after another sham check-up, declared the *already dead* as dead!

Wrote the death certificate and returned to the clinic to attend to the waiting patients.

The question arises: Did I do wrong? Did the declaration of death an hour or more after the actual death really matter? I don't think so. Considering the amount of trouble saved for the household, I felt it was the right thing to do.

❖❖◆❖

A Sacred Duty or a Sinful Neglect?

Some years ago, I used to get help from a surgeon who lived and practised close by. The setup he had was good for minor procedures but not for major surgeries.

One morning I saw a patient who was in severe pain around his anal area, which made him sit on one half of his bottom. And seeing me smile at the way he sat, he said, "You are laughing, you don't know what it means to have pain there," pointing to his posterior.

The smile was quickly replaced by concern, and I made him strip and had a close look. The man had a small abscess [collection of pus] next to the anal margin, an extremely painful condition. What he needed was a simple procedure of draining the pus.

I sent him to this surgeon, with a note requesting urgent help.

An hour later the patient came back. I was happy with such prompt attention and thought he had come to thank me. Instead, the patient said with irritation in his voice, "Please, Doctor, send me to some other doctor. Your friend is *no good*; he spends more time doing his prayers than attending to patients."

185

I agreed to send him elsewhere but was curious to know what had transpired. So, I asked him.

He said, "I went there and waited in his waiting area with other patients. Your friend came, went to his room, and came out with a burning joss stick and proceeded to perform a *ritualistic prayer* to each of the god's photos he had hung in the waiting area. I got cheesed off. He should be attending to us first and do his prayers at home. I lost my patience and confidence in that man and decided to come back here."

So, he went to another surgeon and got the abscess drained.

The surgeon in question became a drug addict and alcoholic and died a few years ago!

❖❖◆❖

B.P: A Perennial Patient

B.P. are his initials. His expanded name is Badri Prasad. I called him BP, coincidentally, as his visits to me caused some anxiety and raised my blood pressure! He did not mind my calling him BP and the name stuck.

It must have been twenty-odd years since BP became my patient. During these long years, he must have seen me hundreds of times—or perhaps I'm *exaggerating*. Every practice has a percentage of patients who have no real disease [or we have not found any] but have plenty of symptoms.

Twenty years back, when he came to me for the first time, it was for a radiating chest pain. The history was so typical that I thought he must be having a heart attack and told him to get admitted under the care of a cardiologist. BP was unmoved. He slowly took out a folder and placed it in front of me. In that folder, I found reports of every test for heart disease available in the city at that time. All tests were normal, but BP continued to have pain.

186

I then said it could be something wrong with his neck that was causing the pain. He took out another folder and gave it to me. It had all the reports pertaining to his neck. There was another folder that had investigations pertaining to his liver, stomach, and gallbladder. All reports were normal. I asked him what medications he was taking. He showed me a list of seven medications, none of which was really required. I told him so and asked him to stop all of them and see what happens.

He came back a week later and said he felt much better and wanted to get his blood pressure checked. After getting his blood pressure checked he would not leave. He requested me to feel his abdomen as he was feeling queasy. That done, he most reluctantly took his leave with the *parting threat* that if things were not alright, he would soon be back.

Things can never be alright all the time. Many minor ailments we are privy to are self-limiting and we don't have to go to the doctor. But BP did. In the course of time, it became a habit. After due examination, I would say, "You are okay," and he would go until his next visit, which was never far away. My worry was that amidst all this normalcy, I would be missing something serious—every physician's nightmare.

Another problem was his habit of consulting all kinds of doctors and then reporting back to me to find out if he could follow the advice given. More often than not I would respond in the negative and he would ask why. Often, this entailed laborious [*to me*] explanation. He would go but would leave behind a lurking doubt in my mind about whether the opinion given by another doctor was right!

Now you must be beginning to understand why I would become anxious with his visits. You are justified in wondering why I put up with him and not refuse to see him. Times without number, I must have told him, "BP, you are wasting your money and time. I cannot help you; please stop coming to see me." His reply always was, "It is my time and my money. Why are you bothered?"

This unhappy situation continued till fate intervened to solve the problem *once and for all*.

BP died some time ago due to septicaemia [virulent infection] unrelated to his myriad complaints. He was seventy-five.

What were my feelings on hearing of his death? Mixed. Relief that I do not have to suffer him and that a troubled life had ended, and some sorrow that I would not see this familiar figure with his huge bundle of medical records.

❖❖◆❖❖

The Futility of Fighting Faith
(Written some years back)

I think it was the late Norman Cousins who said that the medicine that is being practised today is frontier science, and there is more that we do not know than what we know. This truth is appreciated more by older doctors like me than by the younger ones.

This is because of the experience of watching some die due to inexplicable reasons and some survive, once again inexplicably. This knowledge has made me, if not encourage, not to discourage patients from seeking cures by alternative approaches such as homeopathy and naturopathy, when there is no definitive remedy available.

But my experience with these has been generally disappointing. I have had a homeopath treating a patient of mine who had tuberculosis of the lymph nodes on the right side of the neck some five years ago. The nodes swelled and swelled with tubercular pus and ultimately gave away with copious discharge of pus which went on for several months before healing took place by scarring. This was how tubercular infection ended in the olden days before the advent of effective chemotherapy.

Of course, the homeopath took the credit for curing her. The patient came to see me a couple of months ago, and this time there were swellings on the left side. I had an opportunity to examine the other side where healing had taken place with scarring. The whole of the neck under her skin was devoid of tissue and there was a healed scar well-hidden in the dimple above the inner aspect of the collar bone, effectively camouflaged by a necklace!

This time too I explained to her as I did the previous time. Thankfully, she agreed to chemotherapy, and she is well on her way to a recovery, and hopefully I have succeeded in getting rid of the germ, and it will not show up elsewhere again!

It is a well-known medical fact that quite a few conditions, especially ones like headaches, backaches, and some mental ailments do well initially, whatever may be the therapy. Allopathy, homeopathy or *anypathy*—they get better, and some get rid of their complaints forever. These are the people who spread the word around about the miracle cure.

Most illnesses are self-limiting, and do not need a doctor to cure them. Herein lies the success of the alternative systems: curing the illness which is self-limiting anyway. Recently I have had a patient who had a huge hydrocele [collection of fluid inside the testicular sac] who was being treated by Ayurvedic medicine. It was only getting bigger and bigger, and when I saw him, it resembled a small coconut!

Sometimes, I do feel I am biased against these systems of therapy as I see only their failures. But recently there was a review article in the prestigious medical journal, *The Lancet*, debunking homeopathy with facts and figures.

So, despite this knowledge, why do I leave my patients to their ways? I don't do this without first trying to dissuade them. But I cannot and will not force them, as often it is of no use, especially in chronic illnesses like asthma and diabetes.

Latest to this list is the ever-growing popularity of Yoga in its different forms. Here again, as a form of relaxation for the constantly active mind, it may be helpful, but curing an existing illness is doubtful. In a recent double-blind study that I know of, spiritual healing was tried against conventional healing in cases of chronic backache but it failed to prove that it is of any use.

People also seek such help as they have no alternative, like those who are terminally ill with cancer, but I am yet to see one recover. All of them ultimately die. But the believers are a different set of people who are brainwashed into believing what they are told. It also gives them a pastime, something to do.

However, the greatest danger in these practices is that they take away the ability to think differently and hinders their personality development. I have seen this happen to many followers of these spiritual healers, godmen, and godwomen over the many years I have spent in the practice of medicine.

❖❖◆❖

The Accidental Saint

This is another story from the past. It must have been more than thirty-five years ago. Poverty and the alcohol habit often go hand in hand. Perianna was a factory worker, and his salary would be just sufficient to run his family if he did not have this habit of drinking.

When drunk, he was a tyrant and wife-beater, and when he was not, he was a very decent person. His wife and two children had to suffer for him and often were very hard-pressed to make both ends meet despite the money earned by part-time work that his wife, Kuppamma, had.

My advice to Perianna was always listened to with respect, with the assurance that he would ensure it would never happen again, and that he was to quit drinking forthwith. Of course, he did not.

Kuppamma would come for minor ailments for her and sometimes for her two children. Often, she did not have money to pay, and I too would not insist that she pay. Occasionally, she would drop in and pay some money and leave.

This was the situation when one forenoon, I heard a lot of noise and commotion outside my consulting room. There were a couple of patients waiting and I saw some men and women half-carrying, half-dragging my patient Kuppamma inside the waiting room.

She was a terrible sight. Her hair was in disarray; she was incoherent and was saying something unintelligible in Tamil. She was screaming at her attendants and asking them to leave her alone. At my request, the two women who had held her tight set her free but sort of stood guard, lest the patient escape.

I took her by the arm and led her inside. She was docile and had stopped screaming. I made her lie down and asked the attendants what had happened. "*Saar*, we heard her screaming and her children running out and coming to our house. We went to see what had happened. She was sitting, pulling her hair and shouting. We felt you would know what to do as she is your patient, so we brought her here."

I asked them where the children were. "In the house," they said. Thus assured, I proceeded to talk to the patient, by now convinced that I was dealing with a hysterical woman. A couple of questions later I came to know the trigger. The hungry children asked her for food; there was very little available, and the children complained of hunger. That made her go berserk.

She just needed reassurance and a tranquilliser, plus some money. I gave her a 10-rupee note and asked her to go and have some food and feed the children. She was quiet. Overcome with emotion, she sat there weeping, and after a while, she and the others left.

Surprisingly, from then on, Kuppamma stopped coming to see me, and I often wondered what had happened to her. The area she lived in was once a village but saw rapid development with new doctors settling in and maybe, she had found a doctor closeby as it often happens, I thought.

Normally I avoid house calls, especially if they are far away. But sometimes it becomes unavoidable. So, when these two emissaries from *Swamy amma* [lady saint] came and requested that I go with them to see this lady saint, I was a bit surprised. I had heard of this lady saint, and she lived nearly ten kilometres away in a developed area where there were many doctors and even a well-known hospital. I told them so.

They insisted and said they would take me in their car and bring me back. I asked, "If that could be done, why not bring her here and take her back after I've seen her?"

They said, "No *Saar*, she has a high fever and is in bed. She has insisted that only you should see her."

This was indeed a strange request. Maybe one of her followers who is my patient has impressed her with my healing powers. So, I took my bag and went with them. After going for a couple of kilometres, the car stopped at a swanky bungalow, and I saw a small, anxious crowd waiting outside. I was escorted inside the house and led to the lady *Swami's* bedroom. Leaving me there the escorts left.

Whom do I see?

My old patient Kuppamma in this *avatar!* Clad in a maroon *saree* and blouse with an orange-coloured shawl draped around her body, she was reclining in an armchair.

She was ill with a fever for some days. Her doctor disciples were treating her to no avail. That was when she thought of her old doctor. I proceeded to examine her and found her okay except for the fever. I prescribed her some medication, and out of curiosity asked her about her becoming a spiritual person and quite a famous one at that.

Her story:

"Doctor, do you remember that day when I was brought to your clinic? I did not know what had become of me to behave as I did. I fed the children with the money and sat in a corner. That evening, two men came with some offerings and fell at my feet. They were part of the group of my neighbours who had brought me to your clinic. They felt some strange feeling, I believe, after seeing me like that and felt that I was different from what they had seen me as before.

"They also told me that my husband who came home drunk was beaten by me with a stick of firewood. This had convinced them that some strange divine thing had taken over me. This news spread and now people come to me with all sorts of problems, and I offer them some advice. They seem to be quite happy.

"My husband has stopped drinking and has become one of my disciples. The children are in college. I am now at peace with myself and happy that I can help persons in distress." And she thanked me for coming to see her.

She called out for her assistant and told her to pay me.

Impressed, I took my leave without accepting a fee.

❖❖◆❖

The Distracted Doctor

There are many reasons why patients leave their old doctor and go to a new one. Normally, when one is used to a doctor, especially a family doctor, to whom one goes time and again, one doesn't leave him or her for another. There must be some valid reason for doing this. Often it is the distance one has to commute to reach the doctor, as has happened with some of my patients.

There was a time forty-five years back when four of us managed an area within a radius of ten kilometres. Gradually surrounding areas developed and more doctors, daycare centres and nursing homes were established and the patients naturally drifted away from us. Did our practices suffer? Not really, as more people came to settle in our area and they replaced the old patients.

Sometimes they left us for other reasons. Unsatisfactory treatment [from the patient's angle], bad manners [like losing one's cool, *as in my case*], too much wait time, not being punctual and the like. Occasionally, however, there are very strange but valid reasons, as you will see in the story I'm going to narrate now.

Mr. Bhasker Upadhyaya is a pioneer hotelier in this area. His hotel had been there some ten years before I came to settle here. He and his family went to Dr. Sriram for all their health problems. I came to know this Mr. Upadhyaya socially as we both belonged to the same clan and hailed from the same area.

This doctor Sriram was a good doctor and had a large clientele. Some patients of his chose me not because I was a better doctor but because I was closer and there was less waiting time in my clinic. No one spoke badly of him.

So, when Bhasker came to see me in the clinic it was a bit of a surprise. I asked him, "How come you are here and have not gone to Dr. Sriram? Is he away, or what?"

Bhasker asked me, "Doctor, when you are feeling the pulse of the patient, will you be talking?"

I said "No, I will be counting and trying to find out if the beats are regular or not, what their volume is and the like."

"But" he said, "Dr. Sriram while counting, asks me, 'Today what special sweet have you made? You need to make your coffee a bit stronger,' and such unrelated matters. How can he count the pulse while talking like this? He does the same when my daughter goes there as well."

We, doctors, sometimes indulge in this kind of shop talk to put the patient at ease, but not while examining the patient. I tried to defend the old doctor and explained that it must have been a one-off incident, both with him and his daughter.

He said, "No doctor, it happens every time and I have lost confidence in him. My cousin and his family are your patients, and they are very happy. So, from now on, we will come to you." And saying so, he proceeded with his problem.

Thus, by displaying his culinary interests, Dr. Sriram lost a patient, and I gained one.

❖❖◆❖❖

6

PENNY-PINCHING

The Miser's Misery

Sukhmal Shanthilal Jain ran a store in the nearby village of Marappan Palya. His store had almost everything one needed other than groceries. From a pen to a torch, and from a safety pin to a hair clip, you name it, he had it. He took great pleasure in bargaining and made you feel that you got an item cheap, and he happily made a profit. He also did his best to save money wherever and whenever possible, which included paying my fee.

He was thin-built, always appeared to be in distress, and wore clothes that had seen better days. With an unshaven face, he would appear in my clinic, usually for some illness or other that afflicted his children.

If he could, he brought the ill boy or girl himself and avoided his wife escorting the sick child. The reason was simple. Unlike Shanthilal, his wife Paro [Parvathy] did not know the value of money [according to Shanthilal] and was a spendthrift. Once he even told me that she had paid me more than he did!

This Shanthilal, like many others from Rajasthan, had roots in some ancestral village and periodically felt the urge to visit his birthplace. This applied to his wife Paro too. In those days, some fifty years back, travel to his village in Rajasthan took four full days. On one such occasion, after visiting their ancestral villages and doing the necessary temple visits, the party returned to the city.

Our Shanthilal, at the beginning of the return journey, bought full tickets for himself and his wife and a half ticket for his eldest son and did not buy any for the last two, as he thought they would pass for under three years of age. He almost succeeded but got caught by a TT [Travelling Ticket examiner] when nearing the city. Despite his repeated entreaties to be lenient towards a poor person, the hard-hearted TT fined him a total of four hundred rupees.

Shantilal's last attempt at bribing him with fifty rupees made the honest official threaten Shanthilal with doubling the fee and, worse, sending him to jail. Our Shanthilal paid the fine and took out his irritation on his wife and children. The party returned home.

The story did not end there. The next day, his elder son Moti started purging. After he went to the loo a couple of times, Paro told Shanthilal to take the boy to see me.

To this, Shanthi said, "What if he goes two or three times? Last time the doctor asked me to give him more water, and he will be okay. For this small matter to go to a doctor, you think I am a millionaire?" Paro felt there was no point in arguing and kept quiet and went to the kitchen to get water, half-covering her face, as was the custom when confronted with one's husband.

By evening, it became worse, and Moti kept having colic pain and kept going to the loo back and forth, non-stop. Now Shanthilal had to act. Cursing the boy as *shaithan ladka* [son of the devil] and other such curses, he brought Moti to see me.

A four-year-old smart boy, Moti had eaten some infected food during his travel, and the result was diarrhoea. I proceeded to examine him, and when it was over, began to write a prescription.

198

Even before I finished writing and was about to tell Shanthilal my fee, he preempted me and told me the story as narrated above, embellished now and then by how he managed to reach home penniless, thanks to that *bevarsi* [tough to get an equivalent English swear word] TT.

You must have got the hang of it. He was trying to impress me so that I would let him go free. He started leaving the clinic, telling his son, "*Chalo, chalo* [come, come, let us go]."

I stopped him and told him, "You have not paid my fee."

He gave me a look that questioned me in no uncertain terms as to how it was possible that I could ask for my fee, having heard his travails and his having no money. He reluctantly paid half the amount and told me that he would pay the remaining amount later. 'A bird in hand is worth two in the bush,' I thought while pocketing his money.

The next morning, whom did I see? The whole family, including Paro. All down with diarrhoea! This time I had the upper hand. I told Shanthilal, "See, I cannot afford to treat for free or for half rates. Now that you have become poor after your travel, I suggest you go to the free dispensary [which was some two kilometres away]." I could see Paro, who was standing behind him, smiling under her veil.

Shanthi started, "What do you think? I may be poor, but I am honest. I will not run away without paying your fee, just that this is a difficult time for me, *etc.*" I would not budge. I upfront told him the fee that he would have to pay for the treatment of four persons. He said, "I will give. I will give," but made no effort to put his hand in his pocket to take the money out. I too kept quiet and stood watching the fun.

By then, one boy's colic worsened, and he had the urge to have a bowel movement. Shanthilal had no option now. Putting his hand in his pocket, he took out the money.

For his misfortune, he had put a *bundle* of 10-rupee notes in the pocket and forgotten to untie it. He quickly turned his back to me so that I should not see the bundle [*too late*] and took out the money I had demanded. After reluctantly parting with it, he left with his family, giving me a parting shot that said, "Are you happy now?"

All of them got better in a couple of days.

Another time, Shanthilal came with a pain in his lower belly. As usual, he had waited for a couple of days before coming to see me. On examination, I found he had a hernia, which I was able to reduce with some difficulty, and his pain instantly disappeared. Shanthilal was very happy.

But I was not. Though I was sure it was a simple reducible obstruction and not one that would lead to complications immediately after, I needed to warn him of the possible future trouble if it got stuck. He heard me with patience and told me, "I am having it for the last fifteen years, it has given me no problem. Why this operation *gipration*? It will not bother me now as it has gone inside."

"If you get operated now, it will cost you a thousand rupees, and if it gets stuck and you go then, it will be five thousand rupees," I told him. When he heard these figures [here I am writing the rates that prevailed around forty years back], he was taken aback and, telling me he would get back, he went his way.

He, of course, did not get back.

A year later, one night, I woke up to the noise of a rattle created by someone knocking on my gate. I hurriedly dressed up and went out to investigate. Whom did I see? Shanthi and his wife Paro. Shanthi holding his belly and writhing with pain, and Paro supporting him.

I got them inside and checked him to find that Shanthi had an obstructed and possibly strangulated hernia. Instead of coming when the pain began that morning, like his usual ways, he had tried his best to push it in, and after making matters worse, had come to me as a last resort.

When I talked about the emergency nature of his problem, he told me, "You must be joking. Give me one injection for the pain, and you push the damn thing inside like you did last time. The pain will go, and I will be alright."

I would do no such thing and told him to go to the government hospital, which was good, and also because he did not have money to go to the nearby private hospital. Hearing this, his wife Paro said, to his utter dislike, "Doctor *Saab*, he has a lot of money. You give a letter to the doctor in the private hospital. I will take him there."

Shanthilal was not happy with his wife, but he had no option but to agree.

So went Shanthilal to the hospital with my letter to the surgeon. I called that surgeon and told him about the patient and his attitude towards money. The surgery was done, and ten days later, Shanthilal came to see me for sutures removal. The cost of the hospital stay was a little more than the estimate. After getting the sutures removed, he said in a philosophical tone, "Doctor *Saab*, poor people should not get this kind of trouble."

I agreed but said that he was by no means poor. He said, "You don't go and believe what people like my wife say. They don't know the reality." Saying this, he left, still trying to prove that he was not wealthy.

Now, after nearly thirty years, his son Bikram Chand looks after the business. He is better than his father in keeping the clients happy. With education and contacts, he has improved the business manyfold and, unlike his father, is by no means a miser.

Old man Shanthilal does see me occasionally to get his BP checked, and he spends time talking about old times. For some reason, the pleasure I get dealing with Shanthilal, I don't get when dealing with his son Bikram.

❖❖◆❖❖

The Doctor, the Dodger, and the Debt

We doctors cannot choose our patients. There are many types: some are quiet, some voluble, some come prepared, and some unprepared; some are anxious, a few calm; some pay well, some not so well, and some, given the choice, would not pay at all!

Mr. Chandramohan belonged to this last group. Fortunately, my practice does not have many like him, and I tolerated Chandramohan because it gave me a sort of *perverse* pleasure to experience the many ways he and his wife tried to avoid paying my fee.

In this game of his fee-dodging against my attempts to secure the payment, let us see who won and who lost.

Chandramohan came with his smart six-year-old son. His son had had a fever for a couple of days. Nothing serious; a dose of paracetamol every six hours was all that was required. Chandramohan wanted a certificate for school.

That taken care of, he made a *show* of searching his pockets for his wallet and, not finding it, told me, "Doctor, I am sorry, I have left my wallet behind; I will settle your dues *next time*." Without waiting for my answer, he and his son left.

Winner this round: Chandramohan.

Some months passed. Chandramohan came with his father-in-law. He wanted me to examine him and review the reports the old man had brought. As he was a new patient, it took some time, and after half an hour, once the examination and review of the records were complete, Chandramohan paid for the consultation.

I reminded him, "You owe me for the last time you came with your son." He feigned ignorance. I reminded him of the boy's fever and his request for a school certificate. His memory was now refreshed. He said, "Oh, that one, a very small consult; we will settle that later." The shameless fellow paid for what he considered a proper consultation and left.

Who won this time? No one.

The game ended in a *draw*, as I was able to collect the fee for the current consultation but failed to recover the previous one.

Another time, Lakshmi, his wife, came. If ever there was a couple made for each other, it must be this one. If Chandramohan is a dodger, Lakshmi is a *super-dodger*. She has a myriad of complaints, talks incessantly, and takes up a good half-hour for the consultation, examination, and prescription writing. Do you think she paid? No chance. She says, "Chandra will come and pay," adding a thank you before she leaves.

Victory for Chandramohan and his wife.

Next time he visited, Chandramohan looked very worried, as his company doctor had told him he had high blood pressure and had ordered some tests. Chandra wanted to know if that doctor's advice was correct. I reviewed the notes and the reports. That doctor's advice was correct, and I told Chandra as much. "Thank you," he said, and without even looking at me, took his leave.

Clear winner: Chandramohan.

Now he owed me fees for three consultations—one for his wife and one for his son, both done several months ago, plus this one, which he obviously didn't think was worth calling a consultation. I was enjoying this game and was looking forward to his next visit.

Don't be under the impression that our Chandra is financially hard up. Nothing of the sort; by prevailing standards, he could be called a rich person. It is simply his attitude. It pains the couple to part with money, especially when it comes to paying the doctor.

It took the flu season and school re-opening to provide the opportunity. This time he came with both sons. He made the younger one sit outside. After the elder one's examination was complete, he called the younger fellow in. He said, "Doctor, have a look at this boy too; he seems to have picked up a cough." This meant that this *add-on* consultation was free. He got away with paying for one consultation.

Winner: Chandramohan.

I couldn't allow him to keep winning this battle. I had to do some serious planning to thwart him and his wife. I began keeping an account of what he owed me. He must have sensed it. So, next time, instead of coming in, he called me on the phone and described the symptoms his son was having.

I was busy thinking about the patient and didn't understand the ploy. He asked if he could give his son paracetamol syrup, as he had some at home. I told him he could. He said he would bring the boy the next morning to see me. The next morning never came.

Winner? Once again, Chandramohan.

The number of times he had dodged me kept increasing. Matters came to a head when he visited me and began to tell me why he had come. I stopped him and told him, "Mr. Mohan, I want to tell you that I have stopped keeping records of visits and collecting the fee later; it has become a problem. According to my records, you owe me for the last three consultations." I then told him the dates, which included the brief consultation for his son six months prior.

He said, "Of course, Doctor, I will not run away, but this time I have not brought enough cash for the three consultations. I will pay you next time."

"Your house is nearby. Leave your son here, go and get the arrears, and settle your dues *now*," I said.

This took him by surprise. He could never have imagined me being so hard-hearted. Adding insult to injury, the little fellow was laughing. Chandra rebuked the boy for his misplaced sense of humour.

He took his son and left.

I thought he would not return. But he did return after a little while, paid my arrears and for the current consult and left.

Who is the winner? I.

He and his family remained my patients and paid their fees promptly from then on. But I sort of missed the haggle of the past with the family!

❖❖◆❖

A Story of an Empty Wallet

This story is from many years ago. I have had my share of tight-fisted patients. Some were really hard up and try to save money wherever possible. There were others who were reasonably well-off but loathe parting with money, especially when it comes to paying the doctor's fees. Mr. R. P. Iyer was one of these.

Why do they haggle when it comes to paying the doctor? There is a saying that people want to see *their lawyer rich and their doctor poor.* There is some truth in this statement.

This R. P. Iyer, after retirement from a well-paying job [told to me by Iyer himself in an unguarded moment; he must have repented later!], built a house in this area and settled with his wife. He was one of the early settlers here. His two sons and

205

a daughter were married and well-settled in different parts of the country. Iyer's house was some two kilometres away from my clinic.

He suffered from diabetes and high blood pressure and needed to see me frequently. If I asked him to see me after a month, he would see me after two months. He always had a valid excuse for not keeping up with his appointments. Most of these were plausible, but one excuse was irritating. This was, "I took the same medicine that you prescribed last time, and I was fine."

For young readers, it might come as a surprise that the consulting fee then, forty-odd years back was five rupees, and a house call was twenty rupees. Even this was reduced in some deserving cases. Iyer would, after his stint with me was over and the time came to pay me, put his hand in all the pockets of his trousers and exclaim "*Ayyo!* Again I have forgotten to bring my wallet doctor; I will pay you next time," and he would make his escape.

He hoped that I would have forgotten about him not paying when he visited next time. As this had happened earlier, I don't blame him for thinking so.

Thus, when he visited me next and proceeded to pay only for that visit after the examination and consultation were over, I reminded him, "Mr. Iyer, you need to pay for the last visit also." Now his expression became painful. He must have cursed this young doctor's elephantine memory, and saying, "*Appadiya?* [Is that so? in Tamil]" he paid.

Another time, after paying he said, "Doctor, you should show concessions to old, retired persons." My reply that his pension was three times what I earned in a month did not please him.

Another ploy was to offer a 100-rupee note, hoping I wouldn't have change and would say, '*Okay, pay me next time*'.

This too had failed.

Normally he would walk the distance, though with some difficulty given his arthritic knee. Once he took an auto to reach my place. I heard a loud altercation between the driver and Iyer. I went to investigate. I found Iyer up to his old trick. The auto driver had no change for his 100-rupee note. I couldn't help but laugh.

I paid the auto driver and before he went, he [the auto driver] said, "What kind of patients do you have!" This raised Iyer's hackles, and he said, "Doctor, see how arrogant he is, and you support these guys." My paying the driver meant supporting the driver, according to Iyer. After the visit, he paid my fee plus the auto charge. He couldn't escape.

Another incident: This time when I made a house call.

When I got the call to visit him at home, I was a bit surprised. Surprised as he would normally come walking and avoided house calls even when he needed to rest at home. This was because house calls meant paying me more money. This time he had a fever and couldn't walk. Another reason was his son who had come from Bombay [now Mumbai] on a holiday insisted that I be called.

So, I went to see him and saw him reclining in a chair, not looking very sick. His daughter-in-law, after seeing me, wanted to make some coffee for me.

At this, Iyer told her, "Doctor drinks coffee only in the morning," meaning thereby she shouldn't make coffee.

I said, "I don't mind having a cup." This did not please Iyer.

He said, "Doctor, you told me not to drink coffee too many times, and you are breaking your own rule."

I smiled and kept quiet.

He had a mild flu-like illness which would take a couple of days to resolve. Now came the question of paying my fee.

Iyer opened his wallet and took out a 10-rupee note. Seeing this, his son who was watching, told his father, "In Bombay, the doctor charges a minimum of 50-rupees for house calls, and here you are paying this doctor too little." Having said so, he took out two more 10-rupee notes from his father's wallet and gave them to me.

This left the old man very unhappy.

He passed away due to a massive stroke at home. I made a house call this time to pronounce him dead and issue a certificate. While doing this, I couldn't help but recollect the interesting times I had with Mr. Iyer.

❖❖◆❖❖

7

THE CHANGING SOCIAL LANDSCAPE

Every Man Has His Price

Marketing is the buzzword these days. Fifty-five years back, when I began practice in this city [Bangalore], there were very few private hospitals, nursing homes, and laboratories. And those few that existed did not feel the need to market their services in the manner that is being done now.

Some of us had a side lab, an X-ray unit, and an ECG machine, and these were quite sufficient to handle almost all of our patients. The notion that 'more labs, more hospitals, more doctors, more specialists will mean more patients' was unknown to us.

Maybe we lost some patients for want of sophisticated equipment [CT and MRI] and procedures [endoscopy, angioplasty, thrombolysis], but saved many despite not having these. Now it is tough *not* to do a TMT [exercise electrocardiogram or stress test or treadmill test] in a young person with indeterminate chest pain or a CT [computerized tomography] in a person with a headache. Adding to this, there is the menace of high-pressure salesmanship.

Let me narrate a recent experience:

That was an unusually busy day, and the lady must have waited a while before coming in.

Smartly attired in a business suit, she said as an opening gambit, "You have a lot of nice patients."

She must have meant well-dressed [*wealthy?*] patients. My reply was a smile.

She said that she represented a diagnostic service provider and went on to explain the various facilities and the services of the many well-known consultants of the city that were available there. So far, so good.

Now came the *acme* of her sales pitch—it was direct and to the point. For every patient sent to them, I would get a 15% commission.

My expression was blank.

She waited for a minute for a response, and seeing that none was forthcoming, she upped it to 20%!

I felt sorry for myself. Despite my best efforts to keep these executives at bay over so many years, they never take no for an answer, and I have this unpleasant job of explaining time and again why they should not see me.

It was now my turn to tell her why I don't take cuts or commissions and thank her for taking the time to come and see me. She looked a bit disappointed but thanked me for my time and went away. I sat back thinking about this widely spreading malady in the profession.

There was a knock on the door and the young woman was back.

"Sir," she said, "I just talked to my Chief; he has agreed to give 25%, and we cannot go beyond that!"

She must have been a firm believer in the dictum, *'every man has his price.'*

My declining even this offer must have made her wonder how and where she went wrong.

❖❖◆❖

The Ballot and the Bottle
(Written some years back)

The citizens of Bangalore are now in the throes of selecting their ward representatives [corporators], who will administer the city for the next five years. This time around, there are two hundred candidates. Normally, one would expect the contestants to be educated, with a flair for social service, administrative ability, and leadership qualities.

However, going by newspaper reports and what I have seen and heard about these candidates, a large percentage of them appear to be slumlords, gangsters, extortionists and undercover dons who have come overground only to contest the elections. Many of them also have the additional qualification of being school dropouts. Their sole qualification for getting nominations from the major political parties is their *winnability*.

Most are well-known in their respective wards, not for acts of gallantry or social work, but for creating nuisances such as extortion, causing disturbances during festivals, organising processions, and bootlegging. It should come as no surprise that many are rowdy-sheeters registered with local police stations. But they all share one additional qualification: money.

This enables them to hire unemployed youth from the city's slums and shanty towns, where the majority of voters live, for election work. One TV channel showed these young men enjoying themselves after the day's electioneering, sitting in happy groups drinking and dancing. Their electioneering involves visiting voters with folded hands during the day and making clandestine visits in the evenings to distribute goodies like clothing, kitchen utensils, cash, and the prince of all gifts i.e., *alcohol*.

Hooch is the term commonly used for illicit liquor sold without a license. This city has a strong affinity for alcohol.

211

Many years ago, when prohibition was introduced [driven down the throats of people] all over the country, Bangalore was the only city that was spared. This city has inherited many legacies from our erstwhile masters, the British. One of them is this habit of drinking.

Depending on the affordability and social class, there are three main types of drinking men [and women]. The first type comprises the economically well-off, who consume high-end premium spirits [Scotch and other imported stuff]; the second, the not-so-well-off, who drink what is called IMFL [Indian-Made Foreign Liquor]; and the last, those from lower socio-economic backgrounds, who drink the cheapest available alcohol, including illicit brews that often result in death due to methyl alcohol contamination.

But across the board, we Bangaloreans love our drink, and come election time, we give free vent to this love of ours.

Alcohol consumers form the majority of the voting public, and once they put forth their demands to the prospective candidates—*stop making impossible promises*, like providing non-stop water and electricity, clearing the clogged drains, and the like, and instead work towards meeting the following demands!

- Provide shelters near liquor shops where inebriated persons can spend the night instead of on the footpaths and roadside, where they are usually forced to sleep.

- In case people are found sleeping in the above unacceptable areas, ensure they are not disturbed by the police or any good samaritans who pass by. This applies to street dogs as well.

- When we are zigzagging our way back home late at night, passing vehicles must slow down and allow us to go our way. We should have the right of way, and not those crazy drivers.

- Policemen should leave us alone and not drag us to the police station and disturb our sleep and pleasure.

- Wives are a *major problem*. They don't seem to understand the importance of alcohol in our lives. They scream and shout at us when all we want is to get our well-earned sleep. Often, we are made to sleep on the doorsteps of our own homes. This must stop.

- Last but not the least, we are the major revenue earners for the government. The excise levy on liquor forms 40% of the state's revenue. All future corporators, therefore, have to work to reduce the duty on liquor, so all of us can then afford to drink quality liquor and need not risk our lives drinking illicit hooch!

❖❖◆❖

A Prescription for Passion

I wrote this story twenty years ago while visiting the United States and staying with my urologist relative near the Canadian border. It was big news then, and I let my imagination run wild, resulting in this published story. Both the *desi* and international versions have been available for years, and thankfully, the predicted calamities haven't happened!

Here is the story, as it was originally written:

The imminent prospect of Viagra's arrival on the Indian drug scene fills me with trepidation. Why am I anxious instead of being happy about the prospect of many of my elderly patients rediscovering their lost fountain of youth? It appears to be effective in 60% of men with organic [physical] or psychological [mental] erectile dysfunction, or a combination of both. Fortunately, it will not enhance the sexual performance of normal men.

So, what is going to happen when sizeable numbers of men start taking this drug? Mind you, one should take the drug an hour before the scheduled performance, and some men wrongly believe that once taken, it will have the desired effect indefinitely!

Most of the wives of these men will be of menopausal or postmenopausal age, and many will have lost interest in active sex, reconciled themselves to its absence, or even be enjoying life without the pestering of a demanding husband. Viagra might disrupt this *truce*, and these women may once again have to yield to their husbands' sexual demands. A number of them will be unwilling and/or incapable of enjoying sex.

This may lead to problems of ageing men chasing wives of other men, younger women, and even sex workers, with all the antecedent social turmoil. The time may not be far off when we start seeing respectable elderly men seeking treatment for venereal disease, and even worse, for AIDS!

Will a warning that those on medication for high blood pressure and/or heart disease may suffer serious side effects, including death, deter such men from using this drug? I don't think so.

For the pleasure of sex, there are many men out there who will not mind having high blood pressure or even heart disease! Their common-sense argument may lead them to think, "Okay, today/tonight I will take Viagra and omit the BP pill; after all, I have often forgotten to take it, and nothing has happened when I have missed!" And have a go and *'hell with the warning'*.

This drug will sooner or later hit the Indian drug market. Incidentally, the real name of this drug is not Viagra but Sildenafil citrate. Like film actresses changing their names, the drug company that manufactures it has given Sildenafil this *glamorous name*, and this seems to have captured, among other areas of the body, men's imagination as no drug has ever done before.

What will happen when it reaches the market? In the United States, it is priced at ten dollars a pill and is considered expensive even by American standards, yet this has not prevented Americans with real or imaginary need for buying it and lobbying for its coverage by their insurance. There were reports of Canadians, for whom it was unavailable, making a beeline across the border to the United States in search of the drug, reminiscent of liquor-starved Andhras crossing over to Karnataka for their IMFL [Indian-Made Foreign Liquor].

Going by these indications, Indian-made or imported Sildenafil is not going to be cheap. I guess it will cost anywhere between 100 and 200 rupees a pill and will be available only by prescription. It will thus be priced out of reach for a large majority of us who are poor. These people may have to agitate to make this drug available in our government hospitals and use their voting clout to impress our MLAs and MPs to address this issue and make it freely available.

I am imagining the scene in Parliament where our ageing MPs, who may have had the benefit of free use, strongly advocate for the free availability of this drug in their constituencies for the needy or even demand a quota to be allotted to each of them for distribution to those they consider in need. Does this appear far-fetched? *Wait and see.*

The remaining, the so-called middle class, who always have to pay for their pleasures or their miseries, will have a problem: how to obtain it, even if it's only for an occasional indulgence, like their half-glass of weekend beer, they will have to go to their doctor and explain their need to get a prescription.

The family doctor, being *the familiar fool he is,* may not take kindly to this request and may even start lecturing about the

215

need, or lack thereof, for sex at his patient's age, and what his wife would think of this sudden urge, perhaps even launching into a sermon on the side effects regarding his heart, blood pressure, *etc.*

Having overcome this—at the cost of a lowered standing in the doctor's estimation—and having obtained the prescription, he goes to the chemist. It is quite likely he will receive an interested look from the chemist, and the precious potion is *at last* made available!

The next step is taking the pill and hoping that his wife will appreciate the long-forgotten advances and respond accordingly. Even if this hurdle is overcome, the million-dollar question is whether he belongs to the 60% for whom it works or the 40% for whom it does not.

Let us say he is one of the lucky ones and belongs to the successful 60%. He may still face the distinct and extremely unpleasant possibility of not only missing his much-needed morning coffee but also receiving a stern warning from his beloved wife never to put her through the experience again.

He will, then have no option but to wait till another potency pill, this time only for women, is made available, and fondly hope that when that happens, he may not have to tell his wife *what* she told him.

❖❖◆❖

GP Gone!

<u>Scene one:</u>

Patient A goes to his family physician and says, "Doc, I have this headache again since this morning."

"When was the last time you had it?" Doc asks.

"Six months ago, and you gave me some pills to take for two weeks, and I became okay and now I have it again."

The doctor refers to the records, quickly checks his [patient's] blood pressure and temperature, gives him a prescription, and tells him to see him if he does not get better in the next two or three days. The patient thanks the doctor and leaves. The whole process takes less than fifteen minutes.

<u>Scene two:</u>

Patient B finds it hard to go to a family physician or does not have one. There are hospitals he can go to, though. He goes to one. He struggles to find a parking place, and after that ordeal is over, he reaches the reception area and stands in a queue.

When his turn comes, the pretty woman [receptionist] asks him, in a monotone, about his problem. He begins describing his headache. She cuts him short and tells him, "*Neurology*" [Hospital protocol: all headache cases are first seen by a neurologist] and names a fee which is collected and gives him a file with a doctor's name on it.

The patient follows the directional arrows leading to the neurology department and ultimately, after several false turns, finds it. Another reception area and another receptionist, a grim-faced one this time, takes the folder, looks at it and tells him to wait for the doctor to come, as he is busy doing the ward rounds.

When his turn comes to see the doctor, it is two hours, and his headache has reached a crescendo. The doctor asks him how long he has had it. He says one day.

"Any earlier episodes?" asks the doctor.

"Yes," he replies.

After fifteen minutes of examination, he is asked to do some tests, which include an X-ray of his face [sinuses] and a CT scan of his brain [Hospital protocol: for all headache patients, these two investigations are to be done].

The patient trudges to the imaging section and waits in the queue. For his pictures to be done, it takes another two hours. He is asked to come the next day to collect the reports and see the neurologist. It is past 3 pm, and the hungry patient with a continuing headache heads home. Seeing his condition, his wife gives him a tablet of Saridon and then his belated lunch. By evening, after a much-needed nap, he is headache-free!

Next day he goes and meets up with the neurologist with the reports and tells him that his headache has now gone. The neurologist prescribes a drug *anyway* and asks him to take it for the next two weeks.

The drug given to patient A and patient B was the same. Patient A spent 150 rupees and only 15 minutes of their time, while Patient B spent 6,000 rupees and wasted two days!

The latter scene is likely to be the norm if the present tendency of directly seeking help from the hospitals continues, as it prevails. The reason why this is happening is the gradual disappearance of family doctors.

I recently attended a CME [Continuing Medical Education] for family physicians. Normally, in such CME sessions, my preferred seat is in the front two rows, where the speaker is more audible and visible, and it is easy to interact if the need arises. But occasionally I prefer the last row. This is when, for one reason or another, I find the speaker difficult to suffer, and a snooze is preferable to the talk.

On one such occasion, occupying such a vantage seat, I had a view of all those rows of doctors seated in front. There must have been about eighty of them. All the heads were either bald or covered with thinning grey. *No black hair at all!* Most were on the wrong side of fifty.

If no young doctor wants to be a family doctor, what choice does the patient have but to become patient B?

Why have the young turned away from family medical practice?

❖❖❖❖

The Joy and Pain of Telemedicine
(Written some years back)

The noxious advent of the COVID-19 virus put an end to all forms of physical meetings some years back. Weddings, religious gatherings, visits to temples, churches, mosques, friendly weekend get-togethers, professional meetings, seminars, and CMEs [Continuing Medical Education]—all came to a complete halt, thanks to this tiny life form with some thirty-eight genes.

I am part of a club of fifteen doctors that meets once a month, and we have been meeting for the past thirty-five-odd years and naturally have become close friends. We tried holding virtual meetings on the Zoom platform, which sort of ended in a disaster.

It was much like a marriage where the bride and the groom marry and carry on in a virtual platform. This may be tolerable for most of you who are computer-savvy, but for us oldies, it was a real *pain-in-the-neck experience!*

I divide our group into two: one old and the other older. Don't be curious; I won't reveal the ages of these two groups. Those of you who know my age can make a reasonable guess as to the age group of the rest of the members.

In the first virtual meeting attempt, I was happy that all were on time. Some faces were visible, and some voices were heard. Often the voice belonged to the children or grandchildren who were trying to coach the old and the older. The cacophony of noise and the blurred images did not contribute to any learning. Adding insult to injury, most did not know how to mute/unmute, and this ended up with many voices speaking at the same time. Amidst all the confusion, I could make out that most of them were trying to share their experiences in handling the COVID-19 situation.

The second meeting a month later was not much of an improvement. So, we agreed to give this up and continued interacting in our WhatsApp group.

I occasionally get called to participate as a speaker and often as an audience in various webinars that seem to have mushroomed since COVID-19 hit us. I have just enough knowledge in managing these, and I am thankful to my young doctor friends who have taught me this know-how. Do I enjoy these webinars? The answer is no, neither as a speaker nor as a listener.

The reasons are many. The most important one is that I miss the physical interaction. When we attend a physical professional meeting, it is not just the topic that we discuss, it is much more. I probably will ask about my friend's health or how his daughter is doing or discuss a problem unrelated to the topic, on the sidelines of the meeting.

This I cannot do in webinars. The *aura* of personal interaction has gone missing from webinars and the now-popular tele-consults. This loss takes away the very essence of learning and even patient management. There is a TED Talk by Dr. Abraham Varghese on why noting down the medical history and doing a physical examination are so important and the damage to the patient if these are missing, as is happening in the United States. I feel the same with these webinars and tele-consults.

One thing I must accept as good in these webinars is that I am at liberty to snooze unobserved, which is tough in physical meets.

One last word of praise, though not as good as a physically held conference, the virtual conference organised by the Kerala chapter of the AFPI [Academy of Family Physicians of India] was the next best. At future virtual conferences, I suggest having a separate space for meeting friends and engaging in some much-needed idle talk [*gossip*]!

❖❖❖❖

Marketing Madness

Ordinarily, if you are watching any television programme, you are spending [wasting] an equal amount of time watching commercials. These try to sell products that we may or may not need in our day-to-day use. I sat through a three-hour programme and counted the commercials that advertised necessary products. Do not be surprised; they formed only ten percent. Most were unnecessary, and some were positively harmful!

Let me list the harmful ones:

Pride of place goes to food products. These range from soft drinks to crisps and chocolates. All contain refined sugar and fat or sugar alone with additives. Packed with easily absorbable calories, they are tailor-made to make you obese, and going by available evidence, predispose you to cancer and cardiovascular diseases [*The China Study*: Colin and Thomas Campbell]. And there are health drinks containing vitamins, minerals and proteins, especially designed for children and to impress young mothers.

Packaged foods, ready-to-eat mixes, and frozen preserved meats are no good for health when compared to naturally available fresh food. But these are aggressively advertised. Whereas the only time you will see a cabbage, cauliflower, or tomato advertised is when they are on display in a supermarket. There the advertisement is for the chain of supermarkets and *not* for the product.

Next in the list are the body lotions and sprays. Human skin produces sweat, and this secretion has antibacterial properties. That the smell or odour is unpleasant is a culturally motivated phenomenon. Of course, you do not want it to crust and irritate the skin, so periodically one has to have a wash.

But removing the sweat and, worse, spraying the skin with deodorants and scented chemicals [with a flock of women rushing after the sprayed man] is positively harmful. This may cause skin allergies and invite other organisms like *Staphylococcus* to colonise and cause furuncles and abscesses, especially under the arm. There was a time when one shot of penicillin would make these disappear, but now this common, garden-variety germ has become a killer.

Skin-whitening creams too have an important place in commercials. This is especially targeted at women. Why it is considered that a woman with pale skin is good-looking beats me. Again, it is culturally driven, and the advertisements only help to keep this myth growing. It is nauseating to see this commercial.

So are hair growth and conditioning tonics. Mostly useless. But look at the number of men and women buying these products. A senior marketing executive once told me that he could sell even a packet of sawdust with the right idea and image. This is true for most of these products. Sawdust is innocuous, but I cannot say the same of these products listed above.

There is an obnoxious advertisement for skin itch in the groin area. This is usually due to a fungus common in the groin area. Though difficult to eradicate, it is easy to treat with antifungals. But to advertise it the way it is done is positively in bad taste.

We are blessed with abundant health-giving sunlight and dark skin to counter the effects of excessive sun exposure. We are not satisfied with this natural protection. We are forced to use sun protection creams. Except when one has sun sensitivity or when there is danger of sunburn, one should not use sunscreens routinely, as it will stop the production of much-needed vitamin D. As it is, we are seeing vitamin D deficiency syndromes in many office-going men and women, especially those who live in flats.

Likewise, when you have a perfectly working vehicle, why do you need a new one? You need it because the television advertisement tells you that your neighbour has one and your wife is goading you to buy one.

This list can go on and on.

My take-home message to you is: if you have a gadget which filters out all the advertisements from the programme you are watching, please use it. Even better, *do not watch television at all*. It will do your mind, body and pocket a lot of good.

❖❖◆❖

Remembering Gandhi, Ignoring his Message

2nd October is Gandhi's birthday, and the country celebrates it the usual way: another holiday to the burgeoning list, with processions, speeches, garlanding of Gandhi statues, a prohibition on alcohol sales, and the like. *Come evening,* all are back to their typical 'non-Gandhian' ways of living.

If there is one country where Gandhian values are practised the least, it is present-day India. Let us take them one by one:

He preached non-violence as the credo of his life. We have become violent and are growing more violent by the day, both in verbiage and action. Our movies preach violence, and our politicians condone it. Mafia dons and *goonda* bosses are given tickets to contest elections by major political parties.

Next in the order of important Gandhian teachings is communal tolerance and harmony. He gave his life for this cause. Many are not aware that he was a deeply pained man at the time of Indian independence. He did not want this kind of independence where men of different religious faiths butcher each other. Now, not only does this intolerance exist but it has extended to different sub-sects and languages. The major political parties, in Gandhi's name, are fostering this, and today the country is deeply divided on communal, caste and language lines.

He preached minimal needs and manual labour. What do you see around now? Conspicuous consumption and possession of wanted and unwanted things. No one wants to use their hands, and this includes all classes of people. Everyone wants a white-collar job. A man who walks wants a bicycle, a cyclist wants a two-wheeler, a two-wheeler owner wants a car, and a car owner wants two of them and better ones. The same applies to money, clothing, jewellery, a house and what have you.

He advocated spinning yarn as the best mode of providing millions of jobs. Today, who wears Khadi? It has become a dirty word as our politicians wear it to show off!

He did not believe in going to temples to prove his piety. But he led the socially-oppressed to gain entry into our sacrosanct temples. Untouchability still exists, if not visibly but in the minds of people.

Gandhi's dislike of alcohol was more due to its capacity to destroy and degrade human life and not because it was intrinsically bad [*it is bad, like too much food*]. In fact, his close followers, Maulana Azad and Pandit Nehru, were not averse to an occasional tot. Where are we now? In every nook and corner, we have a liquor shop, and hooch is freely available.

He advocated, practised, and preached personal and environmental hygiene. We have the worst sanitation and environmental pollution in the world.

Of course, he had his quirks. The major one was his advocacy of celibacy as a method of limiting family size, and he was against family-planning methods. I am sure he would have changed his views had he been alive today. He probably would have agreed to industrialisation wherever it was required. He would certainly have objected to the loot of our natural resources. Had he been alive, he would have objected even to the export of stones, let alone mineral ore.

So, year after year, we celebrate his birthday and venerate him. But follow his teachings, *we shall not, or will not*. As one of my good friends said, half in jest and half mocking my stupid idealism, "He is irrelevant in today's world."

❖❖❖❖

Conversion Rate

This heading should not lead you to assume that I have suddenly become an economist and have started thinking about the conversion rate of the rupee against the dollar or have become an evangelist dedicated to converting heathens to save them from hell. I am writing about what a doctor friend told me about conversion rates related to a corporate hospital.

My friend is one of those *rare birds* who tries to follow medical ethics. His hospital outpatient work is busy, as he is good at his job and in his approach to the patients. He and I have become friends over the years, and he occasionally confides in me and seeks counsel.

Recently, his hospital's chief called him over for a chat, and during the course of the talk, gently reminded him of his *conversion rates!*

He had a chart in front of him which gave the year's figures of the number of patients my friend had seen as outpatients and the number of admissions he had made. Compared to the previous year, the admission rate had come down, and this, from his point of view, was not good, and my friend was advised to improve his admission/conversion rate.

I have grown old watching the changing medical scenario in urban India. Thirty-odd years ago, doctors held the positions of hospital chiefs, and these were the beginning years of corporatisation of health. Now it is the finance managers with MBA qualifications who become hospital chiefs, and their method of management is how much profit a particular input shows at the end of the year. The input may be *a respected physician or a sonography machine.*

The hospital chief is likely to be a much younger person than the doctor who is responsible for patient care. If I were in his position, I would congratulate the doctor for having reduced the admissions while seeing a greater number of outpatients.

Hospitals are not factories that produce consumer products. These are institutions that manage sick patients, and if a sick patient can be managed as an outpatient at much less cost, it is a service to the patient and indirectly to the community. If the same patient were to be admitted and treated when he could have been managed without admitting him, it may be beneficial to the hospital, but it is unethical!

This is not an uncommon practice, and there have been many occasions when I have given advice contrary to that of the hospital consultant who had advised intervention. And very rarely has such advice from me been proved wrong.

What should doctors, who are at the mercy of the hospital owners, do in such situations? Many are forced to compromise their values and stay on, as quitting the job often means a major drop in their income.

What did my friend do?

He *quit*.

❖❖❖❖❖

The Honour Game: Indian Rules

Honour is a much-used [or abused?] word. This can be interpreted as self-respect, self-esteem, a feeling of being correct, and the like. It also depends on what society at large perceives as honour. Two separate incidents that occurred some years back made me think of these definitions of honour.

An official of BBMP committed suicide by hanging after it was found that he possessed assets disproportionate to his known income. A case was filed by the state's anti-corruption bureau against him. BBMP stands for Bruhat [big, extended] Bengaluru [Bangalore] Mahanagara [huge city] Palike [governing body]. Bruhat can also be interpreted as *unwieldy*,

227

which it certainly is. Bengaluru is the vernacular version of the rather nice name of Bangalore. With the city going berserk with its huge and rapid expansion, the work of the already existing and rather inefficient and corrupt civic body has enormously increased and so has the scope for corruption.

In today's India, it is socially accepted and even honourable for one to be corrupt. Until recently it was so, as long as one remained undetected. Now it has come to be accepted and even applauded if one is caught because it indirectly proves the man's worth!

If another government agency thinks that a particular officer is worth investigating, does it not mean that he gets an official recognition of his worth? It should not come as a surprise to see so many known offenders going about as though it were a privilege to be investigated! More often than not, they are let off after lengthy and fruitless court proceedings, which only adds to the vicarious glamour surrounding them.

It is like gentlemen leaving the top two buttons of their designer shirts open to exhibit their sternotomy scars after undergoing coronary artery bypass graft surgery. Getting coronary artery disease, and more so getting operated on by a famous cardiac surgeon, has become an honour. So, corruption is like a prestigious disease and the investigating agency is like the society cardiac surgeon.

The same news report said that his fellow officers sympathised with him, saying that he [the concerned official] had asked for voluntary retirement [so that he could possibly go undetected with his *honour intact!*]. Even the chief of the investigating agency expressed his sympathy for the now-deceased official.

So, all-round sympathies for a person who killed himself instead of going about with his head held high. Maybe after a few years, he would have had all the charges dropped for lack of evidence! So, this was indeed a rare individual who felt guilty for having been found out! Indian society has been reduced to this miserable state of defining honour.

In the other incident, a couple was killed by the villagers because they dared to marry. What was their crime? They belonged to different castes and thus committed a crime, and the villagers felt *honour-bound* to kill them. You do not believe that this happens in a country that claims to be developing and in due course wants to be a superpower!

Caste and communal identity are primeval, especially in rural India. It is a cursed bond between individuals and families which is held sacred, and anyone who violates this goes against this bond. For persons like me, it is difficult to understand this mindset, but I have known people who may not be indulging in such acts but speak sympathetically, much like the colleagues of the corrupt official who committed suicide.

This scourge is one major factor which will not allow India to become a superpower. Have we done nothing to overcome this? We have—*on paper*. The Constitution guarantees everyone the right to live with dignity. But how can one if the social fabric is like this?

In our own time, there have been persons like Dr. Ambedkar and M.K. Gandhi, and some years earlier reformers like Sri Narayan Guru and Jyothi Rao Phule who crusaded against the evil of casteism. But as one can see, there has not been any sweeping success, and this primordial disease continues to destroy the country.

So, the honour for these villagers is to keep and safeguard their identity. They are not much worried about inefficiency, bad administration, corruption, sloth, dirt *etc.,* which are all around them. Even if these worry them, they do not excite the same fury as the caste transgression does.

229

Next come the honours that are periodically bestowed upon individuals and organisations by the other organisations and the government. Here the definition of honour is recognition. Next only to power is this need to be recognised. Whether or not one deserves to be recognised is not important, as long as the stamp of recognition comes from appropriate quarters.

The Indian government, both at the centre and state, every year honours persons who have rendered services in various fields of activity. Politics is one such activity and bureaucracy comes only next to it in vying to get the honours.

The nation's highest honour, *Bharat Ratna* [Jewel of India], has been so misused that not so long ago, to appease one provincial government, it was given to a *long-dead* Chief Minister of that state!

Similar are the affairs at the state level. One of the persons I know, a social worker, came to know that the state government was considering honouring him. He became so depressed that his name would be associated with so many undeserving persons if he accepted the honour. He heaved a sigh of relief when his name was found missing from the list.

Many professional bodies too indulge in this. Sometimes they do it to buy favours. If they need a big donation, it is natural to catch a wealthy person and entice him with an honour. Or if there is a troublemaker, buy his support by honouring him with a false citation. The recipient, in most cases, will not object to the nonsense written on the citation and the memento.

So, my friends, in today's India, *honour* has many and varied definitions and explanations.

This was written fifteen years ago but remains true even now.

❖❖◆◆

The Bitter Pill of Privatisation

The Indian government seems to have washed its hands off in providing healthcare to its citizens. Going by the evidence of measly allocation of funds in the budget for health and its acceptance of corporate hospitals to provide healthcare to its employees, the trend is firmly set that we are going the American way.

What is going to happen to the existing health infrastructure, the vast network of primary healthcare centres, and secondary and tertiary care hospitals? If the present trend of encouraging corporatisation of medicine continues, it is inevitable that these institutions will gradually go to seed and one day will altogether disappear.

Imagine the situation of excellent institutions like AIIMS [All India Institute of Medical Sciences, Delhi] PGIMER [Postgraduate Institute of Medical Education and Research, Chandigarh], NIMHANS [National Institute of Mental Health and Neurosciences] and Jayadeva Hospital in Bangalore deteriorating and becoming places where only the destitute go!

Nations are spending a considerable percentage of their GDP on providing healthcare. As the population ages, healthcare costs are going to rise and India is no exception. But is neglecting government-run institutions and encouraging private clinics and hospitals run by corporate and health management funds the right way of providing healthcare? Far from it; it is the *worst way*, especially for a poor country like India.

Some of you who are not Indians may wonder when I use the word 'poor' to describe India. What you read or hear about India in the news and electronic media is all about the doings of the 10% of Indians who have done well for themselves. This 10% is what the corporates are interested in. This 10% consists of the upper middle class and the rich.

231

Our politicians [even at the grassroots level] and bureaucrats belong to this class. They are supposed to use the health facilities of the government. Hardly anyone does this, and all of them, with rare exceptions, make a beeline to corporate hospitals when they fall sick or even for their routine health checks. If the top echelons of the government have no confidence in their institutions, how can one expect ordinary citizens to have any confidence on them? They too will and have to go to these privately-run institutions.

With increasing play by the private sector, falling ill has become a risky proposition. Let me explain why. As the private players are mostly businessmen, venture capitalists, and health management funds, the end point of their venture is to make money. They are not doctors who are supposed to think of patients' welfare first and money next [many doctors, too, are becoming *money first and health next* thinkers].

They think of the maximum and quickest return on their investment. If the investment is on a building, they will look at how much a square foot of the building will earn; if it is a bed, then how much a bed will earn; or if it is human in the form of a doctor, how much this doctor will earn for them. That is how they look at each item as a money earner.

Let us say the expected return on a bed is X amount in a year, and the year-end sees that bed earning less than X, then the hospital administrator is pulled up, and he, in turn, will pull up the doctor. The doctor who is so pulled up for not providing the hospital with enough business will either have to quit or adopt methods that his famous Hippocratic Oath forbids him to. Most doctors are not, in the real sense, businessmen to begin with, but they *become* one due to this kind of pressure.

So, what happens is this: when a patient goes to a corporate hospital and sees the doctor, the first likely thought that comes to the doctor is *how much I can get out of this patient* and not what might be wrong with the patient. This attitude, I am sorry to say, is widespread and leads to lots of unnecessary investigations and procedures and needless hospitalisation.

The sucker is the hapless patient. If he belongs to a middle- or lower-income group, these institutions will make him feel that death would be preferable to the torment of raising sufficient resources to meet the expenditure that a hospital stay brings on.

This fear has led to the mushrooming of the health insurance industry. This is another sordid story. Between corporate hospitals and insurance companies, there appears to be a cosy relationship. It is not uncommon to hear the hospital receptionist asking the victim whether he is insured or not.

If he is uninsured, the smile of the receptionist is likely to be replaced by a frown. This is because he is likely to opt for a less-expensive bed and, at the time of discharge, haggle, ask for a concession, create a scene, or as happens occasionally, *simply abscond!*

❖❖◆❖

Spectator Medicine?

Some sixty summers back we medical students learnt the nuances of clinical medicine mostly at the patients' bedsides. The patients generally were from poor socio-economic backgrounds and did not mind a group of enthusiastic students poking their abdomens to feel the hernial orifice or repeatedly placing the stethoscope on their chests to hear heart murmurs. These ward rounds were held in all clinical disciplines.

Ward rounds resulted in a particular student or students being assigned to get the required tests done and do the follow-up. This involved collecting stool and urine samples, drawing blood, and for senior students, performing pleural and peritoneal taps and other minor procedures.

It also fell on us to take these samples to the lab attached to the wards or to the pathology department and to collect the results when due. This often involved ferrying not only the samples but also the patients. This kind of activity resulted in gaining knowledge not only about the diseases but also about the other aspects of patients, such as their socio-economic status and the why and what of their illness progression.

Thus, by the end of the final year, most of us would have imbibed not just knowledge about the illness but also some of the practical skills described above. During the housemanship year, these skills were augmented, and it was not uncommon for a house surgeon to independently perform surgeries such as hernia repairs, circumcisions, vasectomies, hydroceles, and even appendicectomies.

If I remember correctly, we were to conduct twenty-five normal deliveries and assist/observe five abnormal ones. These were *necessarily done* as, in those days, there were no postgraduate students to compete with, and the hands of the unit's senior houseman and the assistant surgeon were always full!

Over these six decades, there have been far-reaching changes in the learning process. First, the number of medical colleges has increased exponentially, and so has the number of medical students. Postgraduation appears to be the norm for most graduates. What was being done by the medical students of my time is now being done by the postgraduate students/residents of today.

With so many medical colleges, many of them privately managed, there is also a paucity of clinical material. Naturally, a patient who has paid money to get admitted to a private ward would not like his or her private parts to be exhibited to a crowd of medical students.

In addition, there is a great dilution of standards.

I learnt that the present-day medical student is *not allowed* to conduct deliveries. Imagine an MBBS graduate who has not conducted a normal delivery being posted to a PHC [Primary Health Centre] and faced with an imminent delivery. I was told it is the job of the *nurse!*

So, there is a major lack of practical training and skill acquisition, and the present-day medical student is a mere observer of the patient and the disease process with no direct involvement. Adding insult to injury, after the final year and during the housemanship year, most students waste their time preparing for the postgraduate entrance test, when they should have been spending time acquiring these much-needed skills.

There are some 40,000-odd postgraduate seats available for nearly 100,000 aspirants. The remaining are left high and dry. Even those who manage to be one of the 40,000 may not get the speciality of their choice, and thus many will end up as *square pegs in round holes.*

One of the remedies to this dismal situation is to strengthen primary care and ensure that an MBBS doctor acquires the basic skills described above. This will result in a more confident young doctor who will not refer patients for the procedures he or she can perform on entering practice.

If primary care and family medicine are given deserved status and importance, this *mad rush* for specialisation of any sort will diminish, and there will be an all-round improvement in the delivery of healthcare in this country.

❖❖◆❖

235

Doctor's Dilemma

This write-up is based on a presentation made at the Bioethics Conference in 2007 and is applicable even today.

A large percentage of our population depends on private medical practitioners for their primary care needs. This is despite there being a well-structured and widely spread network of PHCs [Primary Health Centres] and SHCs [Sub-Health Centres] in place. It is beyond the scope of this paper to describe the ills besetting this network of health centres and why people don't choose to seek help in these centres.

General Practitioners [GPs] come in different hues and colours. They include practitioners of varied systems like *Ayurveda, Siddha, Unani,* Homoeopathy, Naturopathy, Electrotherapy, Hydrotherapy, Reiki, Acupuncture, several kinds of Yoga, and the like. Some of these combine their craft with the dispensation of allopathic drugs. If you include chemists who also dispense advice and medicines, you would not be very wrong. All these provide some sort of primary care.

This paper is confined to the working methods of doctors who practise the allopathic system and who have a basic MBBS degree. In this paper, I have tried to analyse why this section of qualified allopathic doctors has failed to deliver comprehensive, affordable and quality medical care.

It is a basic principle that when a cheaper and more effective drug is available, it should preferably be used by the oral route unless there are specific reasons for not doing so. This rule is generally *not* followed. The reasons are primarily the patient's belief that an injected drug is more powerful than the oral one and also their willingness to pay more.

Doctors put in no effort to dispel this belief and, in fact, exploit this by obliging the patient. The cost of injectables is much higher than oral drugs, and the cost of care thus goes up. Many doctors run unnecessary intravenous drips, and the reason is the same. Demand for X-rays, ultrasounds, CT and MRI scans, and many lab tests is far more than the actual need and, again, is driven by commercial rather than clinical considerations.

With the advent of private players into the healthcare scene, urban India is witnessing a boom in institutions providing healthcare. These laboratories and hospitals are competing for the custom of the paying Indian. Doctors are enticed with monetary and other inducements to refer patients. It is common knowledge that this *cut practice* is widespread, and it adds to the cost of healthcare.

It is also a medically known fact that yearly medical examinations [package deals] as screening methods, when indiscriminately applied to all and sundry, are a huge waste of money and another reason for pushing up the cost of care.

Pharma companies and medical men have always been cosy bedfellows. One encourages the other to the *detriment* of the patient. When one can carry out a decent family practice with about 200 drugs, where is the need for 10,000-odd combinations and brands of drugs that are available in the market?

Pharma companies, equipment manufacturers and hospitals sponsor doctors' CME [continued medical education]. These meetings can be local, in another town/city, or even abroad. Depending on his or her use for the company, the doctor's travel, stay, and even entertainment are taken care of.

The sponsor naturally expects, and in fact gets in return, prescriptions, use of branded equipment, and referrals to the hospital. Those who do not want to enter into such relationships often find it hard to organise professional meets or participate in one. That there are still a few doctors left who have survived is a fact that surprises me.

Are these facts not known to the consumers? Of course, they know, or are coming to know. This is one of the reasons why they no longer hold us with the same degree of respect that they did thirty years ago. Physical assaults and increasing litigation are the direct outcome of this perception that we are exploiters.

Why are we unethical? The answers are many. A combination of the prevailing socio-economic scenario and the compulsion to *keep up with the Joneses at any cost* is one of the reasons. Add to this the basic human quality of greed and the inability to accept a low-profile life in a society that seems to respect only the wealthy.

Add family and peer pressure, and we have a tailor-made situation for practising unethical medicine.

The only silver lining is that society is becoming more informed. Hopefully, the informed citizen of the future will seek out honest doctors, *if they exist*, and will be able to get the profession to mend its ways.

❖❖◆❖❖

Woods, Water, and Well-being
(This article was written in 1999 and is still relevant)

Two isolated yet related events made me write this article. The first was a tucked-away news item in a newspaper that said that the central government had issued instructions that henceforth bamboo is to be preferred to wood in making furniture required for use in government offices. The other was my reading the proceedings of a symposium held in December 1998 at Rishi Valley on environmental problems.

The government order on the use of bamboo was with the intention of saving wood and thereby trees which are felled legally or illegally all over the country to make furniture and fittings, newsprint, and for use as fuel. Vast areas of forest have disappeared to meet this demand.

The universal use of tables and chairs and wooden cots in middle-class Indian homes is a comparatively recent phenomenon. About seventy-five to one hundred years ago, we managed with cotton *durries* and cushions and used reed mattresses for sitting and sleeping.

The use of chairs for sitting has brought in its wake some problems such as stiff backs and hips. In a sample survey, fifty men and women from middle-class backgrounds were asked to squat from a standing position and get up without support. That most of them failed this test did not come as a surprise. This is one minor example of the effect of the use of furniture on health.

The larger issue of cutting trees on a large scale is much more dangerous. Cutting trees results in the washing away of the topsoil and silting of our rivers, which overflow their banks and inundate vast areas of land with loss of cultivable land and create swamps that breed mosquitoes, and you know what happens when the population of mosquitoes increases.

There is a resurgence of malaria, filaria, encephalitis, and dengue fever. There is also an increase in the incidence of cholera, typhoid fever, and gastroenteritis. This is due to the contamination of drinking water with sewage, which is common during floods.

You hear of inadvertent trespassing of whatever little wildlife there is onto the human habitat. This is because of the destruction of their habitat, partly due to encroachment and partly due to the destruction of forest cover and disappearance of feeder species of plant and animal life.

Bamboo furniture is *not* going to solve the problem. Large-scale cutting and use of bamboo to make furniture is also not the answer, as naturally growing bamboo groves are a link in the ecological web of the forest.

The ultimate solution lies in changing our lifestyle and going back to the way of our forefathers. Our homes then will not have to have wood-based products. Metal can be a better substitute for wood and maybe less damaging ecologically.

Destruction of plant cover, which includes forests, has serious long-term economic and health consequences. Rendering the land fallow will mean desertification with no economically feasible agricultural activity, resulting in less grain production and starvation. Malnutrition-related illnesses are very common in our country. Malnutrition causes all kinds of illnesses, including that major scourge tuberculosis.

To sustain minimum nutrition standards, we need to increase the grain production. We have so far done this by taking recourse to introducing hybrid high-yielding crops with ample supplementation of the soil by chemical fertilisers and keeping the pests at bay by using liberal doses of pesticides. This has proved a very short-sighted success and has had disastrous long-term consequences. These pesticides and chemicals have already got into our systems, and the result is that we are seeing an increase in the incidence of hitherto unknown illnesses and an increase in the incidence of cancer. The land enriched with chemicals will not sustain plants for long, and we will be in for a major disaster if these practices are continued.

The only viable solution is to use organic natural manure, for which we need animals and plants and, above all, an abundant supply of water. Many parts of our country that once sustained verdant plant and animal life are now fallow. Large areas of such land can be reclaimed not with Western technology but by following methods indigenously developed by our pioneers.

The efforts of a single man, Rajinder Singh, have brought about an agricultural revolution to 650 villages in Rajasthan. What he did, millions of others can repeat. He simply observed the natural flow of rainwater and built check bunds to slow the rate of flow and made this water collect in small and large percolation tanks. This made the water table rise and charged the wells which were hitherto dry. This primary phenomenon of availability of life-sustaining water makes all the difference to the lives of our people, from one of poverty and misery to one of at least minimum sustenance. This will also arrest the flow of people to towns and cities in search of livelihood.

Rishi Valley is another such example. What was once barren land of dust and rocks has been successfully greened with immense economic benefits to the villages around. The same result can be seen in the work of Anna Hazare at Ralegan Siddhi in rural Maharashtra.

Once a villager becomes self-sufficient in food, his and his family's health improves, and he will listen when we talk about family planning, sanitation, nutrition, etc. An empty stomach resists all attempts at progress.

Thus, health is linked to nutrition which is linked to crops which are linked to the availability of water, which is linked to plant cover, which is linked to soil retention which is linked to us not cutting trees.

All of us will be forced to realise that natural resources do not exist for man *alone*, and this manipulation of nature that is going on the world over to serve the interests of humankind will only invite disaster.

When this simple truth is understood by us and our governments, then humans will start repairing the damage to the environment and reduce their consumption, and nature may forgive the injuries that she has so far suffered.

If this does not happen, humans are on their way to *self-destruction.*

❖❖◆❖

Ceremony and the Servant

Our lives are full of ceremonies of one type or another.

There is a ceremony when a woman becomes pregnant and another when she has advanced some months into the pregnancy, and of course when she delivers the much-awaited baby. Then comes the naming ceremony for the baby. It is not surprising that the perpetrator [husband] is given no role or plays a minor role in these events. This shows how our ancestors viewed conception, pregnancy, and childbirth; the woman who carries this happy burden for nine months is respected, suitably honoured, and rewarded. This process goes on until one's death and even after!

Then there are ceremonies associated with the worship of our numerous gods and goddesses, and each requires a different set of ritualistic procedures. All the above-mentioned ceremonies are confined to religion.

But our penchant for ceremonies is not confined to our religion; it extends to functions held where no religion is involved, such as constructing a building or a dam or repairing a tank when the government is involved.

Before taking up any construction project, an inaugural function is held. This is done on an auspicious occasion [even government buildings are begun after consulting astrologers for this auspicious moment]. This goes by the name "foundation-laying ceremony". A stone plaque with an inscription gives the ultimate use of the building and lists all the dignitaries present on the occasion, along with the date.

Our towns and cities are replete with these abandoned mementos where the intended construction was never completed! They, however, make useful perches for our omnipresent crows and provide a *good rub* for the stray cattle.

In some buildings, you find more than one plaque! Do not be surprised. Each time an expansion takes place, the process repeats! Our government servants want spacious, well-appointed chambers. Even our messengers and attendants want the dignity of a chair and desk. This means a constant need for additional space. There is a continuing construction activity to build office space.

Kindly do not be under the illusion that work gets faster with the provision of additional space. On the contrary, it is delayed. More employees mean the files must move several notches further. More notches mean more delay. It is said that a common Indian is getting throttled by reams of bureaucratic paperwork. Is it any surprise why it is so?

There is a huge [but beautiful] structure in Bangalore called Vidhana Soudha, where legislative business is conducted. We disgruntled citizens call it *Nidhana Soudha*. *"Nidhana"* in Kannada means slow!

There is a prominent plaque displayed in the Vidhana Soudha with the legend, "Government work is God's work!" This is true. The government [meaning those who work for the government] is God. Government workers in India are called government servants. They should instead be called Sons of God, thus a privileged class.

Abraham Lincoln, who said government is of the people, by the people, and for the people, be *damned*.

In modern India, the government is of the government servants, by the government servants, and for the government servants—and *not* the other way round!

❖❖❖❖❖

243

From Hunter-Gatherers to Hamburger-Grabbers

Man domesticated animals and plants [animal husbandry and agriculture] around ten thousand years ago. Until then, he did not know when his next meal was and where it would come from. Most of his food needs were met by gathering wild fruits, edible leaves, flowers, tubers [edible roots], small life forms like ants, flies, moths, and larger life forms like fish, birds, rabbits, deer, and occasionally bigger animals.

At that time, the food was eaten raw. Cooking, the earliest form of food processing, came into being later.

Until the advent of the Industrial Revolution, man ate unprocessed food. Gradually, over the past three hundred years, the food that we eat has undergone a gradual change from an unprocessed, mostly cereal-based diet to a mostly meat-based diet. This is true in Western nations and less so in Eastern nations. The idea that a meat-based diet is healthy, and a cereal-based diet is not healthy has taken deep roots in our thinking.

If you look historically at how chronic diseases like diabetes, hypertension, ischaemic heart disease, cancers and autoimmune illnesses have evolved, one can see a more than causal relationship to these changing food habits. In societies that eat more grain-based, mostly vegetarian diets, the incidence of these illnesses is much less.

Even in these societies, one sees these more commonly in the affluent sections than in the less affluent. Take one example: breast cancer. I have rarely seen breast cancer in poor women, whereas I have seen this in many women in mid- and high-income groups.

Why are we facing a sudden epidemic of diabetes in our country? The answer is in the changing food habits. There is a sudden increase in the consumption of processed, ready-to-eat food. People are also eating more than what is needed for them. Forty years ago, seeing a fat youngster was a rarity. Today, every other boy or girl is overweight. *Too much food is poison.*

Adding insult to injury, there is hardly any exercise. We are obsessed with the scourge called the automobile. Our life revolves around this 'convenience'. That wonderful mode of transportation, the bicycle, has almost disappeared from our roads. Even the poor no longer cycle to work. They too are becoming victims to chronic diseases and diabetes is not uncommon in the urban poor.

In the earlier era, when men walked or cycled to work and women spent time washing, cleaning, preparing food without any mechanical aid, they kept good health. There was no television [TV] then, and people did not sit staring at TV [aptly called the *idiot box*]. Those who watch TV could be called idiots.

Instead of changing our dietary habits and going back to a grain-based, occasional or no-meat diet with little or no processed food, we seem to be *hellbent* on increasing our intake of ready-to-eat food.

The food industry is a major player in keeping our bad habits growing. Advertisements for crisps, oils, butter, spreads, cheese and meat burgers, pies, biscuits and confectionary, beverages, health drinks *etc.*, bombard us day in and day out.

Even we doctors do not spend time trying to change the dietary habits. We are more interested in treating the illness after it occurs than preventing it. Preventive medicine and epidemiology hardly have any takers.

Therefore, my friends, if you want to remain healthy and enjoy life, change your eating habits. Eat plenty of fruits, vegetables, and whole grains; limit your intake of dairy and meat products; exercise for an hour daily; and avoid watching television.

❖❖◆❖

Flock of Sheep

The Medical Council of India has recommended an increase in the number of seats in the medical colleges, and this is to help meet the need for doctors in the country. The human resources ministry also seems to think that by allowing or forcing the IITs [Indian Institutes of Technology] to double their intake, they will meet the demands of industry and will help the socially and economically weaker sections to get access to these premier institutions.

Will increasing the numbers and starting new professional colleges without caring to increase the infrastructure [buildings, equipment, and personnel] bring about the desired result? The answer is *no*, and one can see this happening in post-independent India.

There is an increase in the number of professionals of all types, but their quality has suffered over the years, as evidenced by the calamities we hear about every day in the media [collapsed bridges, train accidents, fires, buildings giving way, patients dying because of wrong treatment].

Some thirty-odd years ago, the late lamented Prof. B.G.L. Swamy wrote the following more out of sorrow than anger:

"I was forced to take double the number of students for the course; this and the number of repeaters made the work of conducting examinations in a decent manner nearly impossible. When I brought this to the notice of the principal of the college and the director of education, the common answer was, 'Swamy, you have to manage it *somehow*.'

"This *somehow* resulted in students taking the examination spilling over onto the pavement. The principal, who came to inspect, seeing students sitting on the pavement, tried to take his ire out on me. I said, 'Sir, what you see inside the room is *some* and what you see on the pavement is *how*.'"

These overflowing, ill-trained students become tomorrow's professionals, and what we are seeing all around is the handiwork of these individuals: a flock of sheep incapable of original thought and deed, capable only of incompetent repetition and blunder.

Who can save this country that is *full to the brim* with incompetence?

❖❖◆❖

In Defence of the Unqualified
(Written some years back)

In recent times, the media has been awash with reports of medical malpractice, and images of unqualified persons handling cases are flashed across the small screen. There were images of a person who is qualified to sweep and clean, giving injections and suturing wounds. There were also reports of doctors performing surgical procedures without taking permission and causing fatalities. These reports received widespread public reaction, mostly directed against the profession.

North India, particularly the states of Bihar, Madhya Pradesh, Odisha, Uttar Pradesh, and Rajasthan is very backward according to social and economic criteria. That is why they are called BMARU [ill] states. In many areas of these states, medical aid is non-existent, and *any aid is better than no aid*.

I watched a programme aired by *Times Now*, a popular English TV channel, that showed a sweeper performing a medical procedure. Instead of getting disgusted, I was very impressed with his performance. He wore gloves, drew the local anaesthetic well into the syringe, injected the wound, and sutured it expertly. There were no nerves at all, and this must have been routine for him.

It reminded me of an incident that occurred many years ago. I was a young subaltern in the Indian Army Medical Corps and was posted to a general hospital. As it was just after a conflict, we had several casualties, and three of us had to do lots of minor and major surgeries. We did have one doctor who was trained in anaesthesia, but he could not be present in three places at the same time. The job of administering anaesthetic was left to two nursing assistants [in the rank of Lance Naik]. They did the job better than I did. They were so well trained!

What is important is not *who* does the job but *how well* it is done. Even well-qualified doctors err. The doctors who did a kidney and pancreas transplant were qualified, and the patient needed it. That it was a high-risk surgery with very high mortality was not appreciated by the relatives. Here lies the crux of the problem. We doctors are poor communicators. We get so engrossed with the problem that we often neglect the human emotions involved and pay a very heavy price.

These days, in corporate hospitals, money too plays its role, and surgeries are often done when there is no absolute indication. One such instance is delivery by a caesarean section.

Therefore, before branding something as demonic and unethical, especially the media, and personalities like Aamir Khan should be careful to understand the realities of the profession in the country.

I have tremendous respect for Aamir, and many aspects of his show were true.

❖❖◆❖

From Sati to Skewed Sex Ratio
(Written some years back)

The recent report on the spate of atrocities against women made me wonder about the possible reasons, and I realised that there are indeed historical reasons, and they are numerous. Let us examine a few:

In present-day India, people can be broadly classified as those living in the plains and those living in the hills. The people living in the hills form a tiny minority and are supposed to be those who were driven to areas beyond easy access [hills and forests] by the Aryan hordes that came into this country some two to five thousand years ago.

Women of the hill people have no problems with their men, as one can see in the northeast, among tribes of Madhya Pradesh, Chhattisgarh, and even in the states of Karnataka and Tamil Nadu. These tribes have traditionally placed women on a different footing than the people living in the plains of India, which comprise the rest of the country.

History is replete with recorded instances of discrimination against women.

The earliest that comes to my mind is Rama's story in the famous epic *Ramayana*. We call this man, Lord Rama, and worship him as the embodiment of everything that is good and great in a human. He is referred to in Hindi as *Maryada Purushottam*. Let us see what his attitude towards his wife, Sita, was, who spent some years in captivity [some DMK historians say willingly!] in Sri Lanka, ruled by the demon king Ravana.

On successful invasion and rescue, Lord Rama returned to the city of Ayodhya with his wife Sita. He, being a noble king interested in the welfare of his people, made clandestine inspections under disguise. In one of his forays, he overheard a washerman make derogatory remarks as to Sita's character

249

during her time in Sri Lanka. This had our Maryada Purushottam Rama worried.

The only way to convince his people that his wife was pure [meaning she had not slept with Ravana] was to make her walk through fire. So, he proceeded to test his reluctant wife with fire. Of course, the ever-virtuous and devoted wife came through this fire test with flying colours and redeemed the suspected honour.

This kind of *horrific* incident is also there in *Mahabharata* [another revered epic], where another king of virtue [except for his compulsive gambling], named Dharmaraja, after losing everything he had in a game of dice, even wagered his own wife and lost. Then this virtuous man mutely witnessed the stripping of his wife in front of an assembly of nobles.

So, men even in those times [two to five thousand years ago] treated women as commodities and not as humans. Women lived and died catering to the whims and fancies of their men.

A woman without her man was considered an economic liability and fit to be burnt along with her husband when he died. This went by the name *Sati*. This barbaric act prevailed till the late 19th century, and it took an English Governor-General, William Bentinck, and an Indian social reformer, Raja Ram Mohan Roy, to put an end to this practice of widow burning.

In present-day India, widow burning is replaced by female foeticide and infanticide, widely practised in many states, with the possible exception of the southern states. Widow neglect is also rampant. There is already an alarmingly skewed sex ratio in many northern states. Single men not being able to find brides is a major problem, especially in a society that treats women as chattels. We are now facing a very serious and dangerous social disaster in the making. Unless society wakes up to this reality, there is going to be a crisis of unimaginable proportions.

Compulsory women's education, preferential treatment, creation of employment opportunities, changes in inheritance and divorce laws that will give women equal rights will help, but the most important thing is a change in the *male mindset*.

Will it come about?

❖❖◆❖❖

Young, Hungry, and Hopeless

When we got Independence, I was a pre-school boy, but I remember those heady days. Nehru was our superhero and could do no wrong. We could not understand why Gandhi was in mourning and was fasting. Now most of us know why.

The woolly-headed Prime Minister was the first disaster the country had to suffer. It is still fresh in my memory when, in the early fifties, the late J.R.D Tata told him to implement family planning, our PM's response was, "Our strength is in our numbers."

At that time, immaterial of caste, community, or religion to which one belonged, one would obey the diktat of Nehru. Such was his influence and power on the Indian people. But he failed to implement family planning in earnest, and our numbers grew and grew. To feed the growing population, more and more land was cleared. To house them more wood was cut, more minerals were extracted, and as the net result, we are today facing an ecological disaster.

Is there any worry among the politicians and the bureaucrats of this country? They seem to believe that *Young India* [more than 70% of the population is below thirty] is the ageing world's salvation. One technocrat, who became a software billionaire and later even became the head of a huge central government project of giving a unique ID to all Indians, wrote in his book that Young India is the future of the world, or words to that extent. That he ended up getting defeated in the general elections is a different matter.

251

What does our new and popular Prime Minister, Mr. Narendra Modi, think? He too is harping on our Young India being the future of this world and makes repeated mention of this in his speeches to the resounding cheers of his mostly young audience.

Now let us see what the reality is. For this 70% below-thirty-years population to be of any use, they should be fed, clothed, housed, schooled, and trained. Even then, it is not possible to employ all of them in our country. In reality, we cannot even provide basic required nutrition to most of this population.

Malnutrition is so rampant that in many states the men and women appear like pygmies. Our primary health facilities are virtually non-existent, and money is spent on building swanky tertiary care facilities, and that too in the private sector. A large part of our rural debt burden is due to the money spent on healthcare provided by private healthcare workers, as people prefer a *private quack* to the PHC [Primary Health Centre], even if there is one within easy access.

Our basic education, let alone professional [any profession] education and training, is in shambles. The government, instead of playing a key role in the fields of education and health, seems to be withdrawing in favour of private players leading to this disastrous situation.

So, we are stuck with an illiterate or semi-literate, ill or untrained, and malnourished young population. What is going to happen to this population? How long will this ill and hungry population keep quiet?

Our present PM reminds me of Nehru. He too was well-dressed and liked to talk to his people. People fell over each other to touch him. I see the *same phenomenon again.*

❖❖◆❖

A Tale of Twisted Tongues

The British, when they were the masters of this nation, gave names as their fancy took them to our towns, cities, streets, homes, flora, and fauna. In this process, the English tongue often mutilated the existing names! Thus, the name Mulagathanni became Mulligatawny, Udhagamandalam became Ootacamund, Veerarajapete became Virajpet, Madikeri became Mercara, Thiruvananthapuram became Trivandrum and Tiruchirappalli was nicely shortened to Trichy.

They somehow did not fully damage Srirangapattana, which became Seringapatam. Thankfully, the latter name did not stick, and the old name is in common use now. Incidentally, Srirangapattana was once a very famous city, being the capital of the Mysore empire under Hyder Ali and his son Tipu Sultan.

Bangalore, sorry *Bengaluru*, was a sleepy village before the British established their cantonment here, and present-day Cox Town and Fraser Town are older than the extensions of Basavangudi and Malleswaram. The old town was just about two square kilometres area confined to a couple of narrow streets, bearing names such as Balepet and Chickpet.

There is also a street called Thigalarpet, named after the community of Thigalas who emigrated from Tamil Nadu in waves in the 15th and 16th centuries. In the famous yearly Karaga festival, the idol bearer is a Thigala youngster.

If one digs into facts from history, one will find these men like Fraser, Cook, Richards, and Bowring did a lot to improve the living conditions in the erstwhile Bangalore, and the names ought to be retained and not changed. What is done is done; we cannot go back to Fraser Town, which has now become Pulakeshinagar, and Cox Town, which has become Sarvagnanagar.

Fortunately, some names have remained, like Assaye Road [in memory of a battle], Osbourne Road, Richards town, Bowring Hospital, and St. Mark's Road. Hopefully, they will remain so.

The naming or altering of names was not confined to towns and cities only. It extended to plant and birdlife too. The peepal tree [*Ficus Religiosa*] is well-known and worshipped by devout Hindus. There is another tree, the leaves of which resemble that of peepal, and the Britisher who observed this called it *Bastard Peepal!* Similarly, he called another tree *Bastard Mahogany.*

The sturdy, darkish-grey kite became the *Pariah Kite*, and the elegant, russet and brown coloured one, the *Brahminy Kite*. I sometimes wonder if the British planter who sat on the porch of his estate home, sipping his gin and tonic water and observing the trees and birds around him, must have thought of these names in a partially inebriated state!

There is an interesting background to tonic water, which is now a popular common addition to gin or vodka and has its origins in the days of the British Raj. Tonic water contains quinine, which gives it that slightly bitter taste. Tonic water came to be used as a preventive measure to control malaria, which most of them must have suffered from, and some had succumbed to.

The other day I was taking a walk and saw a signboard on one of the side streets of Domlur. It bore the name of Erapalli Prasanna, the legendary off-spinner of the sixties who lives nearby. This I thought, was *apt.*

❖❖◆❖

Rashomon Effect
(The source is unknown; it was a forwarded message.)

The forty-year-old gentleman was in deep distress. His wife was rubbing his left shoulder in a bid to alleviate his pain. Within the last forty-eight hours, he had met three doctors [specialists, to be precise] and undergone an ECG, echo, MRIs of his shoulder and neck bone, and a battery of blood tests. The wife's hands were overflowing with the prescriptions, bills, and lab reports.

Being an IT professional, he had often been suffering from neck pain. Three days previously, the pain had started shifting to his left shoulder and arm. Naturally, he googled his symptoms, which indicated the possibility of an imminent heart attack. The couple had rushed to a local doctor who performed blood tests and an ECG and sent him to a cardiologist.

The cardiologist thought it could still be a myocardial ischaemia [insufficient blood supply to the heart muscle] and performed an echo test and a blood troponin test [a protein, levels of which help in the assessment of a heart attack]. It turned out to be normal, but to be on the safe side, he prescribed low-dose blood thinners and cholesterol medications and advised him to get an orthopaedic opinion.

The pain was excruciating, and the orthopaedic surgeon being a specialist in keyhole surgeries, suggested that it could be a tear in the shoulder tendons since the patient was a diabetic. He performed an MRI of the shoulder, which was equivocal. He gave him some more medications and suggested he meet a neurologist *just in case* it could be a nerve problem.

After examination, the neurologist too thought it could be diabetic or viral neuropathy. He advised a few tests and an MRI of the cervical spine. Finally, it turned out to be a slipped disc in the neck bone [cervical spine], and he landed in our net.

What we see here is a common healthcare situation these days. Every specialist sees the patient and his symptoms from his specialised, *narrow* perspective. The clinical notes, investigations and management are tailored to the doctor's specialisation. This is what I would state as the *Rashomon Effect*.

Rashomon is a famous movie directed by the celebrated Japanese filmmaker, Akira Kurosawa. In this film, a murder scene is described by different witnesses from their individual points of view. All the views were different from one another, but they all believed that they were speaking the truth because it was indeed true from their own perspective.

Similarly, every medical specialist has his or her approach towards the patient, typically focused on the system in which he or she has specialised. Upper stomach pain is seen as oesophagitis by a gastroenterologist, angina by a cardiologist, and costochondritis by an orthopaedic surgeon. If we look at their clinical notes and examination findings, it will match their diagnosis since their mind is blinkered. The specialised mind fills the gaps with their previous observations, knowledge about their organ system, and *myopic training*.

With increasing super-specialisation, the patient is not seen *as a whole* but as an affected organ system. The specialist of the organ system falls prey to the Rashomon effect and explains the patient's symptoms from his or her perspective. It is difficult to avoid this in the near future since general practitioners are on the wane now. Unless the medical community talks about this issue, it might reach tremendously dangerous proportions.

What did we do for this patient? We prescribed posture correction while at work, neck stretching exercises and taking five minutes off from the sitting position every hour to do simple neck and shoulder stretches. He followed this regimen for two months and felt much improved. He needed no surgery for his slipped disc.

❖❖◆❖❖

Drowning in Drugs
(Written some years back)

The pharmaceutical scenario in India can be described as an ocean full of fish, of which only a few are edible. The medical profession can be compared to a skilful fisherman who knows which of these are edible and which are not. The patients are those who are ignorant of the ocean and the fish and keep eating inedible or useless fish because they do not know the difference.

There exists a huge number of worthless drugs in the market, and most of them sell. The famous, or infamous [as some are inclined to say], Hathi Committee, which made recommendations many years ago, identified a 100-odd drugs as essential for the practice of modern medicine. This recommendation has been given a *decent burial.* This is the fate of most such honest reports in our country.

One estimate is that there are more than 10,000 drug formulations in the market and more than 1,000 drug companies peddling these! I may not be very accurate in my figures, but they give you a general idea of how many players are involved and what a powerful lobby they constitute.

Let us now consider the common problems faced by our people. Anaemias with or without vitamin deficiencies, infectious diseases of all types, diseases such as high blood pressure, diabetes, heart disease, asthma, cancers, various pains and aches form most of these. All these can be adequately managed with drugs recommended by the expert committee.

257

Let us take one example of tonics. I don't know how this word came into common usage by the patients, industry, and the profession, but on this one word depends a multi-billion-rupee industry. A tonic is something that is expected to pep you up or make you feel stronger.

It is a common experience for doctors to be asked by a patient to prescribe a tonic. Will the doctor say that there is no such thing as a tonic that gives the patient strength and thereby risk losing a patient? *No fears*: most professionals, with honourable exceptions, oblige the patient with one.

I must recount a personal experience here. Years ago, on a visit to my granduncle, I found him taking two spoonfuls of a well-known brand of that useless tonic every day. Knowing that he could ill afford such wasteful expenditure, I felt compelled to tell him so. He told me off and said in no uncertain terms the efficacy of this tonic and that he owed his longevity to its continuous consumption over forty years. The old man is no more, but the brand is still alive, and millions of Indians must be *swearing by it!*

If these are medicinally useless, then why do patients take them? When they say they feel better, are they lying? Sadly no. In medical parlance, there is a term called *placebo*. A placebo is something that will result in some benefit even though it contains nothing aimed at such a benefit. The profession and the industry are more dependent on this placebo value of most of the formulations than the real drug content.

It is known that the wonderful organ brain produces substances called endorphins that are literally like morphine in their chemical structure. Morphine is an opioid derived from the poppy plant and has pain-relieving and pleasure-giving properties. Endorphins do the same.

If given by a doctor to a believing patient with a strong suggestion that he will be better, the brain will release these endorphins, and the patient will feel better. And the same result can be achieved by giving coloured, salted, or sugared water at a fraction of the cost! Only the patient should not know, otherwise he or she may not produce any endorphins.

Treating many of the major health problems of the nation is not difficult. Let me give two examples to illustrate my point:

Hookworm infestation and the resulting anaemia are responsible for a lot of ill health, especially in rural India. To eradicate hookworm, one has to take a single dose of a wormicide and daily tablets of iron for two to three months. The cost of the whole treatment for three months will be less than one hundred rupees. I regret to say that usually the patient ends up paying much more than this because of his faith in tonics and doctors not educating the patients.

Not long ago, two drugs were available which were cheap and effective against iron deficiency anaemia. One was called Ferrocelate, which contained enough iron, and a hundred pills would cost less than ten rupees. And a number of doctors used this to benefit poor patients. Today this brand, which was selling well, has been bought over by another company and is being sold at twenty times the cost.

Another useful formulation was called Macrafolin iron B12. This was also available for around ten rupees for a hundred tablets. Today it is no longer available in the market. There are hundreds of compounds, attractively packed, containing the same iron and vitamins but selling at exorbitant rates.

Doctors prescribe, pharma companies sell, and the poor sucker of a patient is forced to buy. These two examples are sufficient to illustrate the social responsibilities of our leading pharma companies.

This brings me to the relationship that exists between pharma companies and the medical profession. With few honourable exceptions, this is a perfect example of 'you scratch my back, and I'll scratch yours'.

Doctors who do not prescribe or dispense do not impress the patient. The patient is like a devotee who goes to the temple and expects the priest to give him something as a token of God's goodwill. It may be something to eat or drink, or it may just be an offering of a flower. So is it with the doctor. A patient will not like to return *empty-handed* after consulting the doctor. On this single fact of patient psychology, a whole industry of worthless drugs has been built.

Pharma companies adopt the latest selling gimmickry to entice doctors to prescribe. They send their representatives to visit doctors, shower them with gifts, organise dinner/cocktail events with the ostensible purpose of introducing new products, and even pay travel [holiday?] expenses for leading or important doctors.

What about the doctors? How do they, who are supposed to belong to an exalted profession, respond to these overtures? I have come across very few who refuse these incentives.

Doctors must be educated and continually update their knowledge and skills. They will have to attend continuing medical education classes every now and then. Who pays to organise these? Do you think doctors pay for their education? Have no such illusions. It is usually the pharma companies who pick up the tab. Occasionally, medical organisations do attempt and charge a registration fee, but this is only to cover part of the expenditure.

Thus, a *sorry situation* exists. Even good [ethical] doctors are dependent on sponsorship for their continuing education. It is a shame that simple luncheon or tea meetings attract few attendees, whereas cocktails and dinners attract a huge number of hungry and thirsty doctors. You normally do not bite the hand that feeds you. And the doctors who attend these meetings ['eatings' as I call them] end up prescribing the sponsor's product. Here I must hasten to add that the promotion is not always for a worthless product.

Can't doctors then organise programmes without the help of these companies? Of course they can, but it will mean spending money, and when there is someone else to do this, which fool would like to? They have so got used to getting sponsorship that it has become difficult to organise any meeting without help from one or the other of these companies or institutions.

There are very few doctors who can withstand this pressure. On one hand, they have patients who clamour for drugs, and on the other, this kind of salesmanship by the drug manufacturers.

The result is a sea of drugs in which the doctor and the pharma companies enjoy their swim, and the *poor patient drowns!*

❖❖❖❖

Watchdog

My friend has a Doberman pet dog. He is peculiar in his behaviour. Unlike the other dogs of his breed, he welcomes guests with a whine and a vigorous shake of his head and tail. When he sees anyone from the household leaving the house, he gets upset and starts barking.

If you consider my practice as home, and my patients as family members, and me as a Doberman Pinscher, you will be able to follow me. Like my friend's Doberman, I too fail more often than not, and you will know why if you read the next few lines.

Most of you watch television and read newspapers, and you meet friends and relatives. The subject of health, doctors, and hospitals is a favourite topic of conversation, as is reading and watching health-related stuff.

Morbid details of someone's illness and death make a very interesting topic of conversation when the ones discussing it are not involved. But there is also a lurking fear that they themselves would be the subjects of such conversation later. And this adds a bit of *morbid spice*. Now comes the question of how then to avoid this fate?

Many believe that periodic testing [called whole body testing in their language] will tell them if they are fit or not. Little do they realise that these tests will only reveal that the tests are normal but will not tell them if they are normal or not. Thus, this rush to get annual or bi-annual tests done is thoroughly uncalled for, and it has become one of my primary duties to prevent my patients from indulging in this foolhardy and expensive venture.

Am I successful? Sadly, no. The media pressure and the false propaganda by the interested parties are so strong that I am like *a poodle facing a pack of pit bulls*.

The other fad is running to consult specialists. This is another foolish and unhealthy activity. We call this compartmentalised medicine. The body is divided into several compartments, and each compartment has a specialist. The heart has one, the brain has one, the nose has one, the stomach has another, and the list is growing every day. As the joke goes, a patient went with a stuck cotton bud in his *left ear* to an ENT [Ear, Nose, and Throat] specialist. That specialist refused to see him because his speciality was the *right ear* and not the left.

It is my lot to see these unfortunates after they do the rounds. A person with chest pain would have gone to a cardiologist [heart specialist], and finding nothing wrong, would then have gone to a pulmonologist [lung specialist], and then to a gastroenterologist [stomach doctor; sometimes stomach illness can cause chest pain], and then to a psychiatrist [if there is no cause that the other specialists can find, then, there must be something mentally wrong with the patient].

And then he deems fit to see, if he is lucky, a family physician. He [the family doctor] may find the cause to be a chest wall injury suffered some months back as the likely cause of the chest pain. This simple fact was missed by all the organ specialists. Had he gone to the family doctor in the first place, he would have saved himself the anxiety, money, and time.

Another issue is the health insurance *racket*. A person who has healthy habits, exercises regularly, and eats moderately remains healthy well into his seventies. So why does he have to take health insurance? He can save up and invest or keep the same premium money instead of losing it every year to keep the insurance company happy. If you are unhealthy, you will not get insurance, or there will be an exclusion clause anyway. Older people who need insurance do not get it, as they run a high risk of illness and therefore are not profitable for the insurance companies. The whole gamut of the insurance business runs on one factor, and that is *fear!*

Recently I had to visit a hospital and spent some time at the reception where the patients are initially confronted. One of the first questions asked is whether you have health insurance or not.

Why this specific question? Will this mean that you get better attention? *Certainly not.* It will mean you go to a separate bracket where your charges will certainly be higher. This is my hunch.

So, I advise my patients to put aside some money each month and invest it. When the time comes when you are ill, needing hospitalisation [which never comes to most, as death comes unannounced for many of us who are blessed], mostly in your old age, you have enough to take care of your expenses. Most insurance companies also have a ceiling beyond which they will not pay. In this game, the insured is not the winner; rather, the insurance company is.

Do I succeed in getting my patients to follow this advice? You guessed it right—I do not.

Then I find a large number of my patients daily swallowing potions of vitamins, tonics, A to Z [there is indeed a brand like that], minerals, health restorative oils, and health foods. Again, all of this is utterly useless stuff.

But do they listen to me? Yes, they listen [to me] but *don't follow.*

What is the solution to these problems in the community? Find a good *watchdog* [family doctor], look after him, and listen to his well-intentioned barking.

❖❖◆❖

8

LIFE'S RICHNESS

A Music Concert

This incident occurred almost forty years ago in a small town in Coastal Karnataka.

A group of music enthusiasts had formed a body to promote classical music. Since the people who reside there have an ear for Hindustani classical music [a form of classical music that is different from the South Indian Carnatic classical music], this is the form of music they organised every month during winter. It was not easy. Organising a concert meant raising resources, and the music lovers were high in their love for music but low in finances. So, generally, it was cheap local talent that was available, and they had to be satisfied with this.

On one occasion, on the day of their anniversary, they decided to get Bhimsen Joshi. Bhimsen Joshi, even in those days was famous but attainable [later the nation honoured him with the highest civilian award, *Bharat Ratna*]. But it meant spending upwards of 20,000 rupees, a lot of money in those days. Without a sponsor, it was impossible to get Joshi.

The richest man in the town was businessman Ganapathi Kamthi. Ganapathi was known to donate funds to worthy causes. A delegation of music lovers went to meet Mr. Kamthi. After the preliminaries, Ganapathi asked the secretary of the organisation a simple question: "Does this Joshi fellow sing devotional songs [Bhakti Geeth]?"

Joshi was well-known for singing *abhangs* [devotional songs], though he did it in a classical style, which was different from the usual form of rendering devotional songs by one uninitiated to classical form of music. There was an enthusiastic, *"Yes, yes, he does,"* from the group, which was indeed true from their point of view.

Ganapathi agreed to sponsor the meeting. But a problem arose. As the chief guest, he was expected to speak. Ganapathi's knowledge of music was confined to the occasional hearing of Hindi or Kannada film music and devotional songs. The organisers told him that they would write down a speech that he could refer to when asked to make his speech.

On the appointed day, there was a huge gathering of music lovers, and Ganapathi Kamthi was well-received, and he enjoyed all the attention he was getting. He was profusely thanked and was asked to speak. Ganapathi may not have known classical music, but he knew how to impress the audience, having spoken at many business meetings. Referring briefly to the written speech, he extolled the virtues of Hindustani classical music and its evolution, praised Bhimsen Joshi, and thanked him for agreeing to give the concert. He got the deserved applause. The secretary escorted him to the front row, where he sat in high expectation of listening to the maestro singing 'Bhakti Geeth'.

The concert began with *raag* [melody] Malhaar. A single line of a Marathi [another Indian language] abhang was taken, and Joshi elaborated on it in this raag for over an hour. There were several instances of thunderous applause, and when he stopped, there was non-stop clapping for more than five minutes.

There was a five-minute break, and the secretary came to Ganapathi and asked him *"Kash Asa?"* [how is it going?]. Ganapathi gave a noncommittal smile. He was just having the beginning of a raging headache. The devotional song he expected had not even begun. After this one hour of 'torture', he could not understand or appreciate the ecstasy of the audience. There was no escape as the next session of the programme began.

Joshi selected the first line of another song and began rendering it in raag Malkauns. Malkauns is a popular raag in Hindustani classical music, and it is like watching a slow-flowing river, and there are not many highs and lows in it. Joshi spent another hour exploring the intricacies of the raag. He did not go beyond two lines of that song, to the utter disappointment of Ganapathi, whose headache by now was raging.

The musician was in his element. The bond between the performer and the listeners was so intense, and the audience were so appreciative, that after he finished this piece, he took another raag without any break, and this time he chose to sing in Bhairavi.

Bhairavi is a raag that, when sung with intensity and emotion, can bring ecstatic tears to the eyes of the listeners. Seeing so many in tears, Ganapathi thought that there must be something very sad about what this *'fool'* of a singer was doing. Upset, he called the secretary over and asked why they were crying. He was told that these were tears of joy and not of sorrow.

Ganapathi's headache now was at a crescendo. He sat with his head held in his hands, and the onlookers mistook it to be his intense involvement.

At last, the concert was over, and the audience gave a standing ovation to Joshi. After the formalities of seeing the performer taking his leave, the secretary came over to Ganapathi and in all sincerity asked in Konkani, the language of Ganapathi Kamthi, *"Kash laglo?"* [how was it?].

Ganapathi brought all his pent-up emotions to the surface and shouted, "You ask how was it [*Kash laglo, kash laglo mantha*], that son of a wh———e pulled and pulled [*thantha, thantha*] and pulled; it is a surprise his throat did not split, and if you ask me another such silly question, I will break your head, bloody waste of money."

He said this with venomous intensity and walked away, leaving the poor secretary dumbfounded.

My friend, the late Gnandev Kamath told me this real-life story in Konkani, and I am afraid the translation does not bring the same flavour as the original.

❖❖◆❖❖

Confessions of a Frustrated Golfer

Mr. S is a fellow golfer and my patient. He took to golf when he was past fifty, and I have been observing his progress [or regress?] since then. Even when he began, he was not very good, as it often happens when you take up a new sport at that age. Except for the walking involved in golf and the swinging of the club attempting to hit the golf ball squarely, he does no other exercise.

As he has grown older, his never-good golf swing has become shorter and stiffer. This is because he finds it difficult to turn his body fully and shift weight from one leg to the other. Most of us ageing golfers have come to accept this as another aspect of the ageing process and continue to enjoy the game.

This is not so with S. He cannot accept that his bad golf is because of his age and stiffness. He came to see me the other day, and his opening remark was, "Doc, I am giving up golf." I kept quiet.

On many a bad day, I too have felt like doing so but have gone back to play. That *infernal game* is like that. No other physical activity [with the possible exception of sex] is as addictive and frustrating as golf.

"I am not able to strike the ball, and when I do it, it is a slice [the ball taking off to the right in an ugly arc]. I have become abusive and ill-tempered; no caddy is prepared to carry my bag; my partners barely tolerate me; and when I go home, I am so irritable that my wife doesn't even want to speak to me," he stopped.

He sat quietly, staring at me. I can understand the turmoil he was going through. Golf is one game where maximum consultations are done with sports psychologists, and in their absence my friend has found me to help him. I knew that telling him that he had become old, and it was natural that his game would deteriorate would only depress him more.

"What do you want me to do?" I asked him.

"Give me something that will make me less irritable; I don't want to lose my temper on the golf course," he said.

"But then, how will it improve your swing? Have you gone and seen the club's pro?" I asked him.

"Yes, I did. Took two lessons. He wanted to correct my twenty-year-old swing, impossible at my age; it was a bloody waste of money," he said.

"Anyway, you have decided to give up golf. Why then do you need medication to quieten you?" I asked.

"I want to give it *one last try*," he said. I gave him a prescription for a minor anti-anxiety drug, to be taken half an hour before the start of the game. I also told him it might cause some drowsiness. He took the prescription and left.

A couple of weeks later, I met him on the golf course and asked him about his golf.

He said, "I am much better, I have stopped using my driver, 3 wood, and long irons [less forgiving of the 14 clubs a golfer is allowed to carry], and my slice is now much less, though my handicap remains the same."

"How is your temper?" I asked him.

"I am paying my caddy twice the amount so that he can put up with me," he replied. This meant he was bribing the caddy to accept his short temper.

"So, is the medicine working?" I asked.

"Yes," he said, "but *not while playing golf*. I take it at night with my evening drink, Doc. Let me tell you, I never had a better cocktail, and I have never slept this well. You should recommend this to your other patients," he suggested.

This left me *wonder-struck!*

❖❖◆❖❖

Feathered Friends & Fairways
(Written some years back)

For several years, until that day in January 2007, I hardly took any notice of them. A remarkably beautiful grey and chestnut-red bird flew in and sat on a branch of a tree close to the tee box [square piece of levelled turf]. I asked one of my regular foursomes, who had some rural upbringing and knew a thing or two about birds, as to what sort of a bird this was. He said it was a crow pheasant, commonly found in all rural areas.

That was the beginning. Interest in crow pheasant led to other birds, mostly heard but rarely seen. My friend would, whenever asked, give a name to the bird we saw in the course of our play. I suspected this was more to *shut me up* than to improve my ornithological knowledge. I soon realised that there was a great variety of them out there that I didn't know about and what I did know was far from satisfactory [even now, after nearly ten years of birdwatching].

Thus began my quest for knowledge about avian life around me. My playing partners attributed my enthusiasm to the *onset of senility*. 'Having lost interest in one form of birdlife due to ageing, you have taken to this form of birdwatching,' they said!

My attempts at informing these ignorant people that this is far more satisfying and rewarding brought forth great guffaws of laughter. One of them began asking me to name and identify the species every time a woman dressed in brightly coloured clothes passed by!

Armed with a pair of binoculars and the bible of bird watchers, Dr. Salim Ali's book on Indian birds, I became an *odd fixture* on the golf course in the mornings. It amused my fellow golfers to see me on the course in a pursuit different from that of golf.

Recently, one of them, in trying to draw my attention away from the bird I was watching, missed his step and fell into a trench. This obviously succeeded in distracting me, and seeing him prone on the ground, I rushed over only to find him not only unharmed but also full of well-meaning [according to him] abuses at me for being responsible for his fall.

On another occasion, two golfers approached me to find out what I was up to. Finding that I was not there to steal their golf balls [easy to mistake in my shorts and nondescript shirt], they became less hostile and warned me of dire consequences if I trespassed onto the course once again, as it was private territory.

Needless to say, they were beginners and therefore did not know that I was also one of them and pretty senior! But I liked their attitude of saving the course from itinerant birdwatchers and other such unwanted elements. Instead of getting into needless arguments, I agreed to abide by their instructions. A few days later, when I wished the pair good morning while playing golf, there was an embarrassed silence, and one of them rather sheepishly managed to return my greeting.

271

It did not take long for me to realise that the book and binoculars were not of sufficient help when it came to the minutiae of birdwatching, especially in identifying small pale-coloured birds. These were also friskier, and it was difficult to hold them in view for more than a few seconds at a time. I needed an expert birdwatcher to assist me in the details. Through a mutual friend of mine, I got in touch with Mr. T.N.A. Perumal.

Mr. Perumal is a gentleman of indeterminate age. He could be sixty, seventy, or even older. Because of watching and listening to birds, he has developed a keen sense of sight and hearing. However, this is restricted to birdsong, and the sight was made clear to me on my very first outing with him on the course.

He was overwhelmed by the abundance of birdlife [sadly, the number and variety have greatly diminished now] and profusely complimented me and the club on planting so many trees and thoughtfully providing the waterbodies—an ideal habitat for birdlife. I prudently kept quiet [the water bodies are intentionally created hazards to make the game challenging]. Next to the first green, there was an area of scrub jungle [no more] with many tall trees. I found this a favourite of many birds, and I proceeded to take him there.

While we were approaching the green, he heard some bird calling, and he stood still. To have a better look, he inadvertently went onto the middle of the fairway [danger zone]. Sure enough, and soon enough, there were loud shouts of 'Fore!' from the foursome who were teeing off. I had to drag him away from the danger.

He was naturally upset at my indiscretion because the bird had stopped calling, and he could not properly spot it and wanted to know why I had to drag him away just because a few people [birdbrains?] shouted. I told him it was the golfer's call of warning. He grunted and said, "Such loud shouts will disturb the birds."

We went to the edge of the out-of-bound fence and spent the next hour or so watching and identifying birds. All the time, while we were talking, I had to keep telling him to keep the tone of his voice down so as not to disturb the players on the green. This seemed to surprise him. Clearly, he thought that birds are more important than golfers, and if the game of golf had to be played, then it should be done without disturbing the birdlife!

Successive four-balls followed one after the other and as many of them knew me, they came up to us and wished me and wanted to know what *mischief* I was up to. Mr. Perumal did not take kindly to this kind of camaraderie between me and these people who have no respect for birds. He did not say so in as many words, but the frown on his face said that.

Later in the clubhouse, I told him that without these golfers, the golf course would not be here, and there would also be no birds. Instead, there would be another concrete jungle [all around it has indeed become one now]. "Yes, yes, but they should play their game quietly without all that shouting," he said, somewhat mollified.

Over the course of about twelve hours I spent with him over two months, we identified and documented more than fifty bird species on the course at the time of writing. I am still at it.

In Mr. Perumal, I met another of those unsung individuals who pursued an interest for the pure joy of it and took pleasure in educating impatient and rather below-average students like me. He is no more.

My near and dear ones have begun teasing me that I've acquired another *wasteful habit*: birdwatching.

❖❖❖❖

Golfing in Hell

This is a story of two people who had committed an equal number of sins on earth. When they died, going by their record, they both deserved to go to hell. But one was sent to heaven, and the other was shown the way to hell. Naturally, the hell-bound fellow objected to this discrimination. He was told that the other man, who was sent to heaven, was a golfer and had already been through hell on earth every time he played golf!

But, looking at my fellow golfers, I often wonder how many of them really deserve to go to heaven. Take, for example, the conscious grave diggers. I am surprised at the furore created in the press some years ago when *Shivsainiks* [members of a political organisation with linguistic and cultural bias], in their misplaced sense of patriotism, dug up the Ferozshah Kotla cricket ground. This is in the national capital of New Delhi, where cricket matches are held.

This kind of digging, on a much larger scale, goes on in hundreds of golf courses. To see pock-marked fairways and pitted greens, thanks to unrepaired divots and pitch marks, is nothing unusual. While the Shivsainiks were hauled to jail for doing what they thought was a patriotic act, golfers continue to dig up *mini graves* all over our golf courses.

Adding to this, there are gentlemen who believe that the fairway is the ideal place to throw away their empty cigarette packets and butts, and the empty, obnoxious sachets that once contained tobacco chew. I am forever surprised that, despite having a caddy and enough storage space in their bags, these *gentlemen* [?] indulge in messing up our beautiful fairways.

Then there are *slow torture specialists*. These are those who come to the golf course more for their leisurely constitutional than for a game of golf. Surely, a leisurely walk in the sylvan surroundings is highly advisable and may even be therapeutic, but my objection is to their taking six hours to walk the 6,000 yards when behind them are guys like me who want to do it in four hours!

One venerable group, all four of them seventy-plus and happily [for them] retired from active life, play regularly on our course. Even caddies hesitate to carry one's bags when this foursome is ahead of you. To add to their slow play, they get into heated arguments, during which they often forget what the argument is all about.

Playing behind them, I was once a mute witness to a long and heated argument and met one of them walking back in a huff. I couldn't help asking him what the argument was all about. He stopped and thought for a while, but try as he might, he could not recollect the reason. He suggested I ask the threesome ahead and satisfy my curiosity, but he declared that he would not play with these characters ever again! True to character and his short memory, the inseparable four were in place the next appointed day as though nothing had happened!

On another occasion, an exasperated golfer went up to them and asked them to speed up the game. He was ticked off, true and proper. When he reached their age, he was warned, he would probably take twice as much time and may not even be able to play the game. An irrelevant reply, but enough to silence the upstart. We, at the time of writing this, do not know how to handle this group. If you have any sure-cure suggestions to make this foursome play faster without unduly hurting them, please let me know.

There are other golfers who think the golf course is the ideal place to have a picnic of sorts. Our club, in its wisdom, has provided kiosks at two [now three] places, and this encourages this. Some foursomes spend time here leisurely imbibing biscuits and beverages and discussing the weighty affairs of the world.

One foursome has taken to sitting on the bench after finishing their repast and being galvanised into sudden activity as soon as they see the other foursome leaving the putting green. On reaching the tee, one is likely to see one of them teeing the ball with the club in one hand and a cup of steaming coffee in the other. No doubt the disposable cup will be thrown on the fairway, causing further annoyance to the next group. As it happens at two [three] places on the course, you can imagine the hold-ups this causes on a busy weekend. Instead of the suffered wait, most of us have also taken to having the not always welcome breaks.

Our club has recently set up a number of toilets around the course. You may wonder why, when we have a clubhouse which has a greater number of toilets than rooms. But when you consider the number of golfers afflicted with weak bladders, who ever so frequently water the trees around the course and were a sight for sore eyes, this additional provision of toilets is welcome. But it has contributed to the delay.

Particularly offending is the golfer's conversation at decibel levels loud enough to be heard throughout the course. Especially annoying are their celebratory shouts after sinking a putt. While I appreciate their pleasure in sinking a long or difficult putt, I do not believe it is a worthy enough achievement to deserve such high-decibel whoops.

Besides, I have on several occasions missed certain putts after getting jolted by these joyous exclamations on the adjacent green. Let me remind these insensitive revellers that golf rules do not permit one to take the putt again.

You may wonder why, despite all this irritation, I continue to torture myself every weekend on the golf course. Well, it is one way of *reserving my heavenly berth!*

This article, which I wrote many years ago, was published in a journal devoted to golf.

❖❖◆❖

Wodehouseana
(Written some years back)

I first read P.G. Wodehouse when I was at school. Then my knowledge of both the language and the society in which the characters created by Wodehouse lived were rudimentary. I only read them to please my English teacher and never understood a word of what he wrote.

I read him again when I was in college, and the results were a bit better. I must have read and reread them many times since then, and now his books are my refuge. Whenever my mood turns sour, which is often, I take recourse to his books and return refreshed.

Many have told me he is a farce. *Of course, he is.* But he makes me happy. He created a new world of farce based on characters drawn from pre-Second World War British society, and the characters have stood the test of time and have never become stale. The stories written one hundred years ago can still make you laugh. One does not have to necessarily go back to that era to enjoy his works. There is no need to imagine the scenario as it is vividly described when the characterisation is done.

Wodehouse was an avid golfer. Another reason for me liking him. He once famously said, "I wasted the first fifty years of my life because I began playing golf only after." All golfers will wholeheartedly agree with this sentiment. Our lives will be barren and purposeless [*exaggeration?*] if this game were taken away from our lives.

He created a character, an elderly retired gentleman who no longer could play golf but who nevertheless waylaid the unwary in the clubhouse and told them stories recalled from his memory. The stories told by this oldest member [Sage] are available as golf omnibuses, and these too can be repeatedly read without loss of flavour.

The outstanding characters are, of course, Bertie Wooster and his valet Jeeves. The related uncles and aunts, friends and acquaintances, churches and clergymen, country houses, and city clubs fill his books. Some characters are outstanding, such as the pig-loving Lord Emsworth and the genteel, poor PSmith.

At present, I am reading another of Wooster stories and about how he is being helped to get out of or prevented from entering holy matrimony yet again. It is fun reading.

Those of you, I am sure, who get occasionally depressed, given the dismal environment [*at least true in India*], will surely benefit if you take up reading him.

◆◆◆◆◆

The T20 Takeover: Good, Bad, and Ugly
(Written some years back)

The dramatic entry of the 20/20 [T20] cricket into the Indian cricket scene and its success made me write this piece.

There is, undeniably, *some good* to be found in the rise of T20 cricket. Many large cities in the country boast well-built, spacious stadia exclusively meant for playing cricket. The spectator capacity varies from 35,000 to 100,000! Except for a few days in a year, most of these facilities remain unutilised or underutilised. With the introduction of 20/20 cricket, most of these stadia have come alive, with spectators jamming the stands. Imagine over 50 matches held over a three-month period! It is a *win-win* situation for the players, the corporate backers, and the paying, cricket-crazy public.

These matches have thrown open the doors to riches for many players who had no hope of making it to the national squad, for many ex-players past their prime, and for many players from other countries who, for one reason or another, find themselves free to take part. Needless to say, *money* plays a very important role in motivating these players to participate in these matches, hereafter referred to as the IPL [Indian Premier League].

India's darling, M.S. Dhoni, reportedly was bought by a corporate house for 60,00,000 rupees! For those who want to know what this was in dollars, the going rate was 45+ rupees per dollar [when this piece was written some years back]. The glitz and glamour are also provided by film stars and business tycoons who have made use of this opportunity to become more visible and thus sell their wares.

Now let me come to the *bad part* of the show:

Test cricket, as we know it, is played over five days, with bowlers and batsmen striving to excel in the traditional manner. However, it seems to be on its way out. The days of the square cut and the drive seem to be over. The sight of a fast bowler running up to bowl, with three slips and a gully waiting for an edged catch, may become a thing of the past for future cricket lovers. In 20/20 there is no place for the slip; one needs to guard the boundary to catch the lofted pull or punch.

The era of Tendulkars, Dravids and Gangulys has given way to others who are mastering the art of innovating a new array of strokes, and such batsmen will rule the game. *Money bags*, and not the discerning cricket lover, will dictate how this game is to be played and who plays it. Genuine lovers of the game will find it tough to understand the new and changed rules of how the game is played.

This shorter version, which ends in five hours with guaranteed results and short-lived excitement, is prime-time viewing, and, going by the ratings, all other channels have taken a beating. Why watch the important news channel when the 20/20 match is on?

The *ugly part:*

The spectacle of a batsman trying to scoop the ball over the wicketkeeper's head and being applauded in the bargain! The sight of a batsman rising on his toes and striking the ball is like hitting a golf ball with a pitching wedge! Such an ugly sight, but an effective stroke in getting runs! The sight of the ball disappearing over the square leg boundary from a ball pitched outside the off stump! *Blasphemy!*

Then there is the less than acceptable sight of men and women behaving like *demented dervishes* in the stands and of players spitting all over the playing area in the full glare of the TV cameras.

But then, these are changing times, and who will listen to the lamentation of an old follower of traditional cricket?

✧✧✦✧✧

Cricket: The Opium of the Masses
(Written some years back)

The game of cricket is largely confined to Britain and its erstwhile colonies. This is one legacy the colonies bear cheerfully and in which they have also excelled.

For many decades it was Australia; Australians were virtually unbeatable in this game.They were also masters in the art of *sledging*. Sledging is a term referring to acts designed to irritate and cause the batsman of the opposing side to lose concentration and give away their wicket. This is a speciality of close-in fielders, especially the wicketkeeper.

Sledging is identified as the hallmark of the progeny of erstwhile prisoners who colonised Australia! Words like, 'You want to sleep? There are better places,' when the batsmen went scoreless, or 'Now you can think,' when the ball, even when the batsman is wearing a helmet, hits them on the head, can disturb any batsman.

Sensitive Indians were particularly prone to this a few decades ago. Now I believe they too have become experts and have taken to sledging in Hindi, which the hapless Australians do not understand and are likely to misunderstand, as happened between two volatile players, the Australian Andrew Symonds and the Indian Harbhajan Singh.

What Harbhajan said to Symonds in Hindi was 'Teri Maa ki...' [Your mother's...]. Symonds heard it as, 'You are a monkey!' The two came to blows, and the umpires had to intervene. The Sardar [Harbhajan is a Sikh] is not by any means a handsome fellow, but Symonds has some simian features, which added colour to the misunderstood 'Teri Maa ki...'. Fortunately, it was misunderstood, as the Hindi curse has *worse* connotations.

In the enquiry that followed, the venerable and much respected Tendulkar, who had heard the altercation, was hard put to explain the meaning! I believe our own skipper M.S. Dhoni is a sort of expert sledger behind the wickets.

Every four years, a cricket extravaganza is held, and it goes by the name World Cup. Over the years, India has taken over as the prime promoter, and Indian companies spend mind-boggling amounts of money on promotion. The centre of cricket and its power is slowly and steadily moving Indiawards.

Going by the record crowds that attended the first match yesterday, which was a practice match and therefore doesn't really count, we are in for a crazy period of six weeks. Incidentally, India won! Thirty thousand cricket fans paid through the nose for the privilege of seeing the two sides fling a ball at each other 600 times! [It is not as simple as that.]

When the British left India, it was a complete severance. Unlike in other countries where many stayed back, in India and Pakistan none stayed. This was indeed a surprise. So alienated were they from the locals that they had no options but to leave. The first Englishman who opted for Indian citizenship was probably a defrocked priest called Father Verrier [read the famous, well-written and researched biography on Father Verrier by Ramachandra Guha]. But many of their habits and institutions survived. The game of cricket is one such.

The other is our Clubs. In most of urban India there are these organisations where friends [members] gather mostly to drink in private [though not entirely true]. These clubs have their own *archaic rules*. Until recently, one of these in Bangalore did not allow women to become members! Even now, you cannot enter some clubs wearing comfortable *kurta* pyjamas. If you enter in a *lungi*, it is possible that an elderly member clad in a suit may suffer a heart attack.

Cricket caught on like wildfire. It suited us very well. We are an overpopulated country with a large number of partially or fully unemployed people. These people have found it great to spend time watching this game for five days. In those days, there was no limited-overs cricket, which ends in six hours. They could sit back, relax, sleep, do nothing and watch the game, in keeping with our *national character*.

With money and newfound affluence, this pastime has become a monstrous obsession and addiction, and the newly-rich cash cows are hellbent on making us all slaves to this game, especially the shorter 50-over and 20-over formats.

✧✧✦✧

282

Cricket and Cinema: The Glue of a Nation
(Written some years back)

I sometimes wonder what is holding us together as a nation. We are so many, and we owe our allegiance to different creeds and ideologies. We are a nation of over a billion people. We elect our leaders rarely based on virtues of honesty and ability but on issues like caste, religion, money, and muscle. This we have been doing for the past seventy years, and it has progressively worsened, and, as you can see from the headlines in our newspapers, we are a poorly governed country. But we have managed to remain as a nation. *How is it possible?*

It could be that these divided loyalties make us realise the larger issues of nationhood and prevent us from destroying democracy. It is like Rumpole the lawyer [*Rumpole Omnibus*, John Mortimer] defending a petty criminal and getting him off so that he remains a petty criminal and carries on and doesn't graduate to serious crime. So, though they are not our best specimens, our politicians, in their own flimsy way, have kept our nation going.

What else is keeping us together? There are two things, and these days I feel these two have contributed more to keeping our identity as Indians going than our politicians.

Let me deal with the first one: It is the Great Indian Cinema, especially Hindi Cinema, popularly known as Bollywood, exclusively produced in the city of Mumbai. Hindi is a language spoken and understood by most of us. There are two types of Hindi movies. One is called commercial cinema, and the other is called art cinema.

Commercial cinema produces the largest number of movies and is viewed by almost all Indians, whatever their allegiance to other interests may be. They may be rich, poor, Hindu [and many sub-classes], Muslim, Christian, Sikh, Buddhist, Jain, *etc.* They all watch this commercial cinema. All commercial movies have a simple formula. They have a story which revolves around heroes, heroines, comedians, villains, and other characters, both evil and good. Ultimately, good triumphs, and the viewer is happy.

There is no real need for our heroes and heroines and, of course, our villains to know how to act. Acting is a *by-product*. What they should know is how to dance, and they must be good-looking and well-muscled. The heroines must be well-proportioned and be prepared to show as much of it as possible. An average Hindi formula movie has at least ten song and dance sequences and the same or a greater number of fights. These will keep the audience spellbound for over three hours.

The art cinema, surprisingly, is *not dead yet*. These are movies that are occasionally made that depict the real India and her struggles. It is, therefore, rarely entertaining. An average Indian does not want to see on the screen what he is experiencing in his day-to-day life. He wants to live in a world of illusion, at least for those three hours. It is no wonder that these reality cinemas rarely make enough money, and that they are still being made is surprising.

What I have written about Indian Cinema is what I think and is not supported by my personal experience, as I am not a moviegoer, having decided long ago that it is a waste of time and money. But my surmise that Hindi Cinema is one of the binding forces of our nation has many takers.

The other is Cricket. Here I can write with some authority, having been an avid follower of the game for the past fifty years. Of all the mad habits the British left behind, such as never using hands to eat food, wearing dark-coloured suits in midsummer, and playing and watching cricket, the last-named has the maximum following.

Few mad Indians still follow the first two. It is not uncommon to see an Indian desperately trying to eat a *masala dosa* with a fork and knife or profusely sweating in a dark suit.

284

But the trait of watching cricket is across the board and is a universal habit. Before the advent of television, this addiction was confined to the playing arena and a few thousands who watched and many more who listened to the running commentary over the radio. Now the viewership has grown so much that it is estimated that one in every ten Indians watch or follow the fortunes of Indian cricket.

It has been attributed to the late Bernard Shaw, who described cricket as a game played by twenty-two fools and watched by twenty-two thousand! Going by his definition, we are a nation of fools, given its popularity. Fifty years ago, there was only one version, which is now called Test cricket. This went on for five days and often ended in a draw [an honourable name for neither side winning]. Drawing the Test match, especially when played between India and Pakistan, was the boring norm.

Though Test cricket still retains its popularity in some quarters, the shorter versions, the 50-over and 20-over cricket, have overtaken Test cricket in popularity ratings. This is because, in these shorter versions of cricket, it is certain that there will be a result, and the game ends in a day or a few hours.

Indian cricket, over the years, has produced some outstanding individual cricketers but rarely a team that won consistently. There were more losses and draws than wins for the team. Individual brilliance of a Kapil Dev or a Sachin Tendulkar does not win matches. It needs a team of good players led by a captain who has qualities of leadership. After Mansoor Ali Khan, who was the Indian team's captain more than forty years ago, we have not had an outstanding captain who won matches for us until the advent of a man called Mahendra Singh Dhoni, two years ago.

M.S. Dhoni, popularly called Mahi, is one of those rare persons who are born to lead. The way he walks, talks, thinks, and acts is that of a leader, and under him, Team India has won match after match in almost all countries. This applies to all forms of the game.

There are some outstanding players, but the credit for knitting the team together and making them play as a unit goes to this one single individual, M.S. Dhoni. It is not an easy job. The team usually has members belonging to different religions, castes, and languages, and they come from all parts of this large country.

In earlier years, we were not well-known for our physical stamina and build. But now the team looks and behaves differently. They no longer appear small either physically or in their deportment. They have no fear.

The two openers we have are small-built men. One of them is Virender Sehwag. Seeing him, you will not believe he can hit the ball that long and that hard. He probably is the best hitter of the cricket ball in world cricket today. One can see the helplessness on the face of the opposition when he cuts loose. There is all-round consternation. He reminded me of the West Indian cricket writer C.L.R. James, who wrote about a West Indian batsman who had a simple philosophy: "I will try my best and see that the wicketkeeper has no job to do." Sehwag once said, "The ball is there to be hit, and I will hit it. In the process, if I get out, so be it."

Then we have Yuvraj Singh, who believed that a ball that can be hit for a four can also be hit for a six. He hit an English fast bowler for six successive sixes in one over!

One outstanding leader can make so much difference, and Team India is now probably the best one-day team in the world. When are we going to produce a political leader of the calibre of Mahendra Singh Dhoni?

End piece:

In a county cricket match, the fast bowler Freddie Trueman was bowling. Reverend David Sheppard was one of the slip fielders. Trueman hurled the ball at the batsman, who edged it. The ball went between Dave Sheppard's legs and sped to the boundary. Freddie gave one of his famous glares, directed more at Dave than at the batsman. The next ball met the same fate. When the over was completed, Dave told Freddie, "I am sorry," to which Freddie replied, *"Not you, your mother should be."*

Another version goes that Dave apologised and said, "Sorry, I should have kept my legs closed," to which Freddie replied, *"No, not you, your mother."*

(Story told to me by a friend.)

✧✧✦✧✧

The Thrill of the Kill
(Written some years back)

In ancient times, Romans would set humans against animals and watch the resulting gore from specially built stadia. Next came the era of gladiators who fought against each other to the merriment of the audience. That tradition is seen even now in the form of bullfighting.

The bulls do not fight; they are killed after being tired from chasing a red cloth being waved by the modern-day gladiator called a matador. Bulls occasionally behave in a wayward manner and succeed in attacking not the red cloth but the matador. This element of danger is what interests the audience, and the ultimate killing is done by piercing the brain of the animal. This so-called bullfight is one of the *most brutal* of sports practised in modern times.

Next in order is boxing, where two humans fight each other. Elaborate rules and gear make this less bloody than killing the bull, but fighters can get killed or maimed for life. The famous Muhammed Ali suffered such severe brain damage that he became a cripple in middle age. But the sport is quite popular, and even the Olympic Games include it, and that too in many categories, depending on the weight of the participants.

Next comes car and motorcycle racing. I just cannot understand the popularity of this sport. If impending death is what one wants to watch and call it a sport, you have a perfect example of this in motor racing. The recent tragic deaths of two young men, one in motorcycle racing and another in car racing, seemed to have heightened expectations and popularity.

In our country, the land of *ahimsa*, a huge track has been built in Noida, and we are going to have this *bloody sport* soon. The likes of Tendulkar, Yuvraj Singh and co. seem to think that they should support this sport by buying teams!

The horse is a wonderful animal. In grace and bearing, I do not think there is any mammal that is as good-looking [including humans] as a horse. What have we done with this animal? We train it to race with a man sitting on its top and urging it to run faster by beating its haunches with a specially-made strap. And thousands throng to watch. Society women use this as an occasion to show off their costumes and headgear. But again, the popularity is partly due to the *element of danger*, where the horse as well as the rider may come to harm.

Of course, there is an element of injury risk in most sports except probably in table games. Most sports require skill, stamina and fitness, and the pleasure gained is the reward of those physical and mental efforts.

The perfect example of such a sport is badminton. One should watch the likes of Dan of China and Wie of Malaysia playing against each other. It is impossible to believe that a human being can be so fit and agile. There is hardly any threat of someone getting killed playing badminton, ping-pong, or tennis.

As sport-loving people, we should stop watching motor racing, horse racing and boxing and shift to watching other sports, *even if it is that sham, twenty-twenty cricket!*

❖❖◆❖

Finding Happiness in Everyday Life
(Written some years back)

This morning the button that anchored my trousers snapped. Fortunately, it happened at home, and no embarrassment ensued. I needed to sew the button back onto the appropriate slot. Though this was no emergency, I felt I should try my hand at it.

My wife keeps a kit with sewing thread rolls and assorted needles. It had been some years since I had done this, and I was not sure if my seventy-five-plus-year-old eyes were up to this job. It was with tremulous hands that I took hold of the needle and thread, and it took me just three attempts to succeed in threading the needle. Sewing the button on was easy. That I was able to thread the needle made me *very happy* at that moment.

Happiness is difficult to describe. In a way we can say it is the opposite of sorrow. Sadness is easy to define, but happiness is not that easy. One can say that it is a state of mind where, at that moment, there is a sense of euphoric contentment. I have experienced this often.

There is a pair of bulbuls who are resident around my home, and they regularly patrol, and part of this patrol includes the shrubs that line my driveway. Bulbuls have a very fruity call, and when I hear the call, I go out and watch them. Suddenly, for almost a week, I did not hear or see them, and I was becoming a bit anxious about their safety. Then, two days later, I heard their call. *That was happiness.*

The other morning, while playing golf, I witnessed a glorious sunrise, and *that was happiness.*

But all these sensations/feelings are ephemeral. Can we make this feeling permanent, even when we are faced with problems, pain, and suffering? I heard a Buddhist monk speak on this subject. According to him, it is possible by meditation, which will rid the mind of negativity and will elevate and educate the mind to experience happiness all the time. Such a mind will be rid of desire, jealousy, anger, and anxiety, which are the basic causes of most suffering.

I honestly do not know if meditation helps or not, but I know this much: material possessions and the desire for such do not bring happiness. On the contrary, they can be the cause of unhappiness.

What about pain? Does meditation help to overcome or lessen the pain sensation? Sage Ramana Maharshi was seriously ill with disseminated cancer, and he was in severe pain during his last days. When asked, he told his disciple, "Yes, the body is suffering, but the mind is not," or something similar. Those who are interested can get more details on his last days by searching online.

I have written in the past about Robert Trent Jones, the all-time great golfer, and the stoic way he suffered the disability caused by syringomyelia. There appears to be a lot more to learn about how the mind controls emotions. It may make good reading to access Norman Cousins' books, *Anatomy of an Illness* and *The Healing Heart.*

❖❖◆❖

Nature's Orchestra
(Written some years back)

Some of us don't need an alarm clock to wake up. Those who are sensitive and know how to listen to birdsong can wake up to their call.

The breeding season for avian life is from March to May, and the first call is often that of the Barbet. The loud *kkttroooo—ktrooooo*, repeated over and over, is enough to wake anyone up. But most don't because they are deaf to bird calls. If one sees the size of a Barbet [about that of a small Myna], one cannot help but marvel at its ability to produce this high-pitched sound. The small Green Barbet has a white patch on the cheek below the eyes and some brownish freckles on the neck. There are many varieties, but the ones you see in and around here are the small green ones.

Some years ago, I witnessed a spectacle of a crow trying to get at the eggs in a Barbet's nest. The alarmed parents were making frantic calls, perched on a nearby tree. They need not have worried, as try as it might, the crow couldn't reach inside the hole and the cavity where the eggs lay! The nest was dug out of the wood from the centre of a cut branch of a tree. The next year, too, they chose the same spot, and the depth of the cavity was just enough to defeat the crow's beak!

After the Barbet's call comes the Koel's. A melodious to shrieky *kuooo—kuooo*, over and over, with the female responding with a rather ugly *quik quik* response. The Koel is easy enough to identify, as the male is a smaller and sleeker version of the jungle crow. The red eye is a giveaway. The female is shy and not as good-looking as the male, with the body speckled with brown and white. The Koels are on the increase, and this I suspect is because of the increase in the crow population. If you are wondering *why*, it is because the lazy Koel drops its eggs in the nest of the unsuspecting crow.

Next to give a wake-up call are the Tailorbirds.

I am not an ornithologist, and neither am I an expert bird watcher. The former needs knowledge of taxonomy, and the latter hours of patient observation, both of which I lack. Therefore, I often make the mistake of naming them incorrectly. This is especially true of small birds like the Warblers [Prinias]. This is because they are so frisky and never stay more than a few seconds at any one place.

It took me a couple of years to make out that the pair of Warblers, who are resident around my house, are indeed Tailorbirds. It is by their song, a kind of sweet and loud *teewity*, that I was able to place them. The other common Warbler one sees is the Ashy Wren-Warbler, which makes a noise like that made by garden shears cutting a hedge—a *chuck—chuck* sound. Another common one is the Plain Wren-Warbler seen among scrubs and bushes.

But the most remarkable one is the Orphean Warbler, which migrates to India, all the way down to Tamil Nadu during winter months, and then goes back to Afghanistan and Baluchistan! It again, makes a *chuck—chuck* sound and, during the mating season, has a melodious loud calling song! It can be identified by its greyish-black top and off-white lower portion. How this bird, which is about the size of a sparrow, flies all the way and survives to breed here is beyond my comprehension.

The other common bird that one occasionally sees is the Robin, which is a black beauty with a small white patch on the side. The female is pale brownish-coloured and is commonly seen with the male. If you are fortunate, you can see and hear the Bush Chat, which closely resembles the Robin. This bird has such a melodious song, the like of which I have not heard. Like the other members of the avian world, the male is far more beautiful [to the human eye!] than the female.

Next comes the Sunbird. You can see this one, which is half the size of a Sparrow, on almost all the flowering trees because it is a nectar feeder [also berries and small fruits] and is usually seen in groups. If you have a Singapore cherry tree around your home, be on the lookout for these birds during the fruiting season.

One must see this bird with binoculars to appreciate the multiplicity of colours and the beauty. A common one in our neighbourhood is the Purple-rumped Sunbird. This bird has crimson, purple, blue, light yellow and green colours. I consider this the most beautiful of the birds that I have been fortunate to observe.

After 7 am, there is no point in trying to listen to the birdsong. The *cacophony* of us humans would have begun by then!

❖❖❖❖

Golden Oriole: A Flash of Yellow
(Written some years back)

There was a time, some ten-odd years ago, when my golf course was next to a wooded area and not surrounded by a concrete jungle, as it is now. The Golden Oriole was frequently seen and heard in those days. The sightings have become rare, and I saw one some two weeks ago perched high on a tree.

I was walking below a canopy of medium-sized trees yesterday, and I heard the distinct song of the bird. Looking up, I saw it. Startled [most of the bird and animal life avoids humans, *justifiably so*], it took off in a yellow blur.

The male Oriole is an orange-yellow and black bird with a thin black eye patch. It is a very beautiful bird. Though locally migrant, they seem to travel quite widely, and, given the

293

migrant character of the species, the Golden Oriole spends winter in the extreme north of the country.

The song is a fluty, short whistle, just like that of the bulbul but a bit more prolonged. Once heard, one cannot fail to recall it, as I did, and I could identify the bird even before I saw it.

✦✦◆✦

The Sandpipers: A Spot of Joy
(Written some years back)

For the past ten-odd years, I have welcomed with pleasure a single pair of this bird each year from January to May. I carried a pair of binoculars with me whenever I went golfing in those days, and despite that, it took me several days before I could definitively identify this bird as a Spotted Sandpiper and not a Common Sandpiper.

They went missing [or I missed seeing them] for the last two years, and when I saw them once again a week ago, it was like meeting some long-lost friends.

Sandpipers are migratory birds and are known to fly from one continent to another. The pair who come to my golf course probably come from Europe or Northern China. The characteristic brown top and white bottom, the bobbing head and tail, and their feeding habits are all characteristic.

Usually found near the edge of ponds and lakes and even on seashores, this class of birds seems to be in no danger of extinction.

I was, and still am, a happy man after I saw them hale and hearty, though I found it hard to explain this to my fellow golfers!

✦✦◆✦

Rosy Pastor

Englishmen whiled away their spare time in pre-independent India pursuing many productive activities. One of them was watching birds and trees and naming them. This was a major contribution to our knowledge of plant and birdlife around us. Among the others was the production of a delightful community of mixed blood called Anglo-Indians.

Rosy Pastor is the name given to a bird [size of a common myna] which has a rose-coloured front with a black hooded head and has a peculiar habit of looking down [appearing to do so]. Imagine a pastor [priest] with his rich robes castigating you for some mischief you have done, and you have the Rosy Pastor. What an apt name!

Rosy Pastors [I don't like the new name of *Rosy Starling*] breed and live in Eastern Europe and migrate to India from September to March. Fifteen years ago, I used to see thousands of them. On one occasion, during the fruiting season, the orange berries of the *Ficus* tree were completely hidden from view by the avidly feeding Rosy Pastors. In the early 1930s, a bird watcher observed that the sky went dark when a flock of Rosy Pastors flew by. Such was their number.

This has decreased so much that I did not see any last year and thought I would not see them this year, either. But I was in for a delightfully surprising experience.

I went golfing the other day to a golf course located some distance away in a semi-rural setting. While I was about to putt on one of the greens, I heard the unmistakable chirp of the Rosy Pastor. Looking up, I saw a row of these Pastors, resplendent in their rose-coloured fronts with blackish hoods raised, chirping [praying, I thought] for my putt to drop into the hole. There were at least thirty of them sitting on the silk cotton tree branch, all looking in the same direction.

It took some pressure from my partners to make me leave that spot. The putt, of course, was missed, with me imagining a row of red-fronted and black-hooded priests perched on the tree branch in supplication. You cannot putt with this kind of imagery disturbing you. The missed putt was *worth the sight*, nevertheless.

Some of you must have heard of the names *Brahminy Kite* and *Pariah Kite*. The Britisher who named these two commonly seen kites must have been well versed with the caste system and the looks of different castes in the country. The colourful white and russet brown kite was named *Brahminy* [Brahmin], and the rugged, dark grey kite, the *Pariah*, though both raptors live on the dead and rotting flesh!

❖❖◆❖

Crows and Sparrows

My friend Dr. S.R. Jayaprakash is not only a good physician but also a well-known wildlife photographer. His knowledge of flora and fauna is much deeper than mine. While I write about what I see around me, he does not. He has commented on the disappearance of the sparrow from urban Bangalore.

The health, or otherwise, of our delicate environment is often judged by the presence or absence of some forms of life. The sparrow is one such example. Sparrows and crows are two birds who have lived with humans in perfect harmony. Why, then, has the crow survived and the sparrow almost disappeared?

Here are some interesting phenomena which are linked to our changing lifestyle. Years ago, this city had many beautiful tile-roofed homes [some relics can still be found in some old localities]. The city also had hedges instead of cemented compounds. These were ideal nesting sites, and it was very common to see hundreds of sparrows living in proximity.

Unafraid and friendly, they survived mostly on grains. People in those days carried grains in hessian [jute] bags, and spillage was common. They also had this habit of spreading grains on mats in the verandahs to dry.

Now concrete has replaced the tiled roof and plastic has replaced the porous hessian.

In some pockets of the city, like Shivajinagar and Lakhmipuram, I have seen sparrows still surviving!

Crows have survived better than sparrows because they thrive on the abundant garbage, which the fastidious sparrow cannot stomach!

Some forms of life and humans have a symbiotic relationship that dates back thousands of years. Dogs and cats have manipulated us to their survival advantage. The same is true of food crops like cereals and grains, not to mention livestock.

Crows and sparrows, too, have lived alongside humans and have depended on us for their survival. There are two types of crows one sees: the house crow and the jungle crow. The jungle crow is larger and lacks the buff-coloured neck of the smaller, sleeker house crow.

Some Hindu castes have a yearly ceremony commemorating their dead forefathers. Female ancestors are not considered worthy of commemoration. This ceremony is confined to three generations to make it convenient. The ceremony involves the offering of cooked rice balls to crows. Crows are considered to be representatives of the three generations of the deceased. Only when the crows eat the offered rice can the family eat. That is the rule.

The house crow, which used to be commonly found around houses, is becoming scarce in the city centre, and the report of a family waiting for *over six hours* for a crow to arrive made hilarious reading. As this ceremony is quite sacred and a must, these Hindu castes have to think seriously about ways to ensure that crows are present.

One way is to keep the crow as a pet, like one does with the parrot, and put up with its *constant cawing*. But would the free-spirited crow accept captivity? Would the crow's unavailability and the resulting inability to complete the propitiation ceremony land these Hindu castes in trouble? The disquieted spirits of three generations of ancestors would probably haunt the living with unknown dire consequences!

Why have the crows become rare in the city centres? One reason may be the garbage collection system that has been in place for the past ten-plus years. It may also be because modern Hindus are giving up the yearly ritual as a worthless ceremony. Or is it because the priestly class of Brahmins who officiated these ceremonies is becoming rare, and therefore there are necessarily fewer rice offerings, and consequently the crows are rarely seen?

Interesting thoughts.

❖❖❖❖

A Fruit Tree and its Visitors
(Written some years back)

My balcony overlooks the backyard of another house. Here grows a sapota tree. *Sapota* or *Chikoo* [*Manilkara Zapota*] is a fruit-bearing tree that originated in Brazil and has spread all over the tropics. In India, chikoo is a major horticultural produce. The tree fruits twice a year, and a well-looked-after tree bears fruit in thousands.

The owners of this chikoo tree are old and cannot reach the upper levels of the tree with ease, and thus lots of fruit remain unplucked. I am ever grateful to them for their unintended generosity. Twice a year, when the tree fruits, it becomes a veritable bird-watcher's paradise.

I have on a previous occasion written about a family of squirrels that have laid claim to the fruits and how jealously they guard them against predators, mainly birds. It was a pleasure to watch the mostly futile attempts of the squirrel family to chase the birds away.

This year, however, they seem to have found that it is a waste of time to chase the birds away, especially when there is plenty of food for all! Another new feature I noticed this year is that all the birds have begun feeding at the same time, unlike in previous years when they took turns.

The Green Barbets came first, and the others followed. This year I was able to watch all of them feeding at the same time. I had not noticed Mynas in the earlier years. This year there were at least ten of them.

The most fastidious and elegant of all the feeders [according to me] is the Koel. This big bird perches next to the fruit and elegantly pecks without disturbing the fruit or letting it fall.

The worst of the lot is the Parakeet. Not only is it very noisy [I tolerate its screech only because it is a bird and a good-looking one at that!], but he is very wasteful. A Parakeet's beak is curved and designed to open pods and eat the seeds, and not to consume ripe fruit. In attempting to eat, he ends up dislodging the fruit, which falls to the ground only to be eaten by the Crow.

The more I see the Crows, the more I am impressed with their intelligence. Earlier I used to see them eating the fruit while still attached to the branch. Now they wait below for the half-eaten fruit to fall to the ground. They, unlike the other birds, are unafraid of us humans and can risk doing this, their easy way to get at the fruit.

The Parakeet [Rose-ringed Parakeet] until recently was a visitor. But now it has become a resident. I was wondering at the unusually prolonged presence of this bird around my home when I discovered its nest! The preferred nesting site is a tree with a dead branch or one with some holes in the trunk. There is a dead coconut tree some hundred yards away, and this dead tree stands some fifty feet tall. This is an ideal location for the Parakeet's nest. I have begun watching these birds sallying to and fro, and by the way they are behaving, there are sure to be hungry chicks in there.

Chikoo is not a fruit for which one sings paeans of praise, unlike the Mango. But it is a great fruit, not only in the abundance of yield but also in taste and structure. There is very little wastage; the skin is thin, the seeds are few, and the rest is delicious flesh. No wonder my avian friends and I like it so much.

❖❖◆❖

Celebration of Life
(Written some years back)

Baisakhi, Ugadi, Vishu—you call it by any name—is an important festival for Indians all over the country. This day is celebrated as the day of beginning of new life, and Mother Earth is thanked for her bounty. This day also heralds spring and a new and hopeful beginning. This is also the birthing season for most avian life and the budding season for plant life. I see this all around, and it fascinates me.

Sardar Khushwant Singh wrote about a tree that he planted in his backyard growing huge, with a canopy of leaves under which he relaxed and enjoyed its beauty.

I observe a young peepal tree undergoing the seasonal change. A few weeks ago, it started sprouting new leaves of light lemon-yellow colour. These gradually turned light brown, then a flamboyant greenish-yellow, and soon will be a glorious dark green. All this happens in a matter of a few weeks. I watch with fascination the early morning sun reflecting these colours and the tree acquiring a rare beauty.

Indians have worshipped the peepal tree [*Ashwath*; *Ficus religiosa*] from ancient times, and there is no village where this tree doesn't occupy a central place in the scheme of things. The embankment built around it acts as a meeting place and social club for the villagers, and the huge crown of leaves gives the much-needed shade in the scorching summer sun.

The abundance of fruit, common to all *Ficus* trees, is heaven for birds. These trees live for centuries. Another famous *Ficus* tree, the Banyan [*Ala*; *Ficus benghalensis*], grows huge and broad and lives for centuries.

My favourite *Ficus* tree remains the common tree known locally in Kannada as 'Goni Mara' [*Ficus mysorensis*]. This too, grows huge, but not as huge as the peepal, has arboreal roots [I have never seen one touching and implanted on the ground like you see with banyan], and has closely placed branches and leaves so the tree is more compact than the others, with hardly any space in between.

It bears enormous quantities of fruit, initially yellow and turning orange-red when ripe. It is a sort of Mecca for birds during the fruiting season. These are common trees planted on either side of roads and also grow in wooded areas. Now, if you are lucky enough to see this tree, it looks from a distance like a green crown of leaves studded with orange and red fruits.

A relative of this tree is *Ficus benjamina*, commonly seen lining the main avenues of the city. These long-lived trees can be found in a few locations in Cubbon Park, near the tennis stadium, and must be at least 200 years old based on their girth and height.

Treewatching, like birdwatching, can be a very satisfying hobby. Unlike birds, trees don't fly away, allowing ample time to appreciate their beauty.

The late Mr. Neginhal, forester, botanist, and tree lover, once said: 'There is no better hobby and pastime than planting a tree and observing its growth.'

❖❖◆❖❖

The Name Game: A Botanical Puzzle

A couple of years ago, I came across a close-up photograph of a Sunbird perched on the branch of this flowering shrub. The commonplace ornamental shrub is found in most gardens, and one of them is next to my bedroom window. It attracts a lot of insect life [bees, in particular] and provides a good perch for birds.

I have placed pails of water, and many birds [including the boisterous crow] come for a drink and, after quenching their thirst, spend time on the branches of this tree/shrub. I have watched with pleasure sunbirds, warblers, bulbuls, not to mention pigeons and crows. An occasional visitor is a kite.

I asked around for the name of this shrub and even wrote to the author of the photograph but could not find out its name. My interest waned, and the matter rested there.

Some years later, my friend and fellow golfer Roger Binny wanted to plant this shrub in his farm and wanted me to collect the seeds or grow some saplings and give them to him. He too wanted to know the name!

The one person whom I should have asked earlier, but did not, was my wife! She said, "I don't know the English name, but in Kannada it is called *Ratnagandhi*." At last, I had a name.

Further research showed it to belong to the family *Caesalpiniaceae*, and the botanical name of the tree is *Caesalpinia pulcherrima*. A tree native to the tropics, possibly imported to India from either South America or Barbados. It has the distinction of being the national flower of Barbados.

There is another Kannada name for it: *Meese Hoovu*. Literal meaning: Moustache flower. A very apt description, if one looks at it from close quarters.

The saplings I provided to Roger matured into full-grown, flowering shrubs on his farm.

❖❖❖❖

A Floral Symphony

In the midst of so much that is ugly in our city, there are these magnificent trees, belonging to two distinct botanical families, giving us immense visual pleasure. With their bloom typically occurring between January and May, these trees are a common sight in any neighbourhood.

The *Cassia* family has one set of trees which have red to pale pink and off-white flowers and another set which have yellow flowers. They are all smallish trees, and when in bloom, the whole tree is one big spectacular display of colour with hardly any leaves visible.

Of the red varieties, my favourite is the *Cassia nodosa*, or pink *Cassia*, and I am fortunate to have many specimens of this tree in the vicinity. They give me a lot of joy even when they are not in bloom!

Among the trees having yellow flowers, the best and the most beautiful is *Cassia fistula*. A few years ago, one evening while trekking in the foothills of the Nilgiris, with the vague hope of sighting elephants near a watering point, I saw this specimen in full bloom amidst dry brown scrubland. The inflorescence has hundreds of flowers drooping downwards, and the placement of each flower is such that it looks like an inverted golden necklace with a broad base and a tapering end. I am at a loss to describe the beauty of the flowers. Imagine the whole tree full of these flowers!

I have not seen this tree in Bangalore, but I was told there are some in Lalbagh. Maybe it is exploited as the fruit and flower pulp is used as a laxative!

Tabebuia is another family which has a fair representation in Bangalore. The ones that catch everyone's eye are the common, stunted, gnarled, misshapen, smallish trees laden with golden yellow bunches of flowers [*Tabebuia argentea, Tecoma*]. When in bloom, there is no leaf, and it is all flowers.

Tabebuia rosea is a big, well-shaped tree with a huge crown of deciduous leaves which make way for pale rose-pink flowers. When in bloom, the whole tree is covered with flowers, and it is a traffic-stopping sight. The trees exhibit a staggered bloom, ensuring a display of flowers over a considerable period.

But the one I like most is *Tabebuia avellanedae*. This is another common and favourite avenue tree, smallish with broad leaves, and when in bloom, the whole tree is magnificently mauve.

Those of you who live in and around my area can see these trees in full bloom on either side of Jeevanbimanagar Road in the month of December. You can also see a number of them arranged in a circle in front of the Public Library in Cubbon Park.

Last but not least, there is the all-time favourite, *Jacaranda*. This delicate tree showers its blue flowers, and the ground underneath looks like it is covered with a blue blanket. The sight of these trees in bloom is unforgettable. A drive along the Old Airport Road, after Manipal Hospital, to the left during their blooming season, offers a view of a striking blue floral display.

The pleasure that these trees give uplifts the spirit. To experience it is pure joy!

✧✧◆✧✧

Nature's Fireworks

Copper Pod [*Peltrophorum pterocarpum*], or rusty shield bearer, is a common avenue tree that blooms in April. It is a large, well-leafed tree and, when in bloom, bears tons of orange-yellow flowers arranged in clusters. From a distance, the tree appears aflame with orange, interspersed with green.

The flower has five thin, wrinkled petals beautifully arranged in a circle around a central bunch of stamens. With hundreds and thousands of these flowers, the whole tree looks remarkably beautiful.

Double Road, which connects 100 Feet Road to ESI Hospital in Indiranagar, has a profusion of this tree on either side. This stretch of the road could have been appropriately named Copper Pod Avenue but has been renamed as Paramahamsa Yogananda Road!

✧✧◆✧✧

9

A POTPOURRI OF PONDERINGS

A Tale of Two Doctors and a Village full of Characters

Sixty years ago, the government, in its wisdom, thought that two months of rural posting during the housemanship year would sensitise the budding doctor to rural medicine and expose him or her to the rural socio-economic environment. The fact that quite a few students came from that environment escaped the attention of the powers behind this stupid move.

The only way for students to take an interest in rural medicine is to make their five-year learning mostly rural-based and strengthen the primary care setup so that most graduates willingly become primary care doctors and hopefully will not hanker for becoming specialists of one sort or the other.

That this experiment has failed to produce doctors willing to work in rural areas has not led the authorities to give up these two months of rural posting and to think instead about changing the entire MBBS curriculum to suit the needs of the people. Even today, most medical students consider this two-month posting as a sort of wasteful punishment. We were the first victims of this folly.

Ramanagara is a small town, and the primary health centre there was chosen for our training in rural medicine. This town then was connected to Bangalore by a single-lane road, some 40 kilometres away. The connectivity was good, as most buses and trains going to Mysore stopped at Ramanagara.

Two of us, Dr. A.S. and I, reported to the doctor at this centre.

That doctor there asked us, "What do you want to do?"

This was strange, as we thought he knew what we needed to do. We told him so. Obviously, he had yet to receive clear-cut instructions as to what and how to manage us!

He thought it best to send us with the ANM [Auxiliary Nurse Midwife] on her field visit, to begin with. Asking us to report the next day, he said, "Where are you guys staying?"

We were under the impression that this was taken care of by the health centre.

He said, "There is no accommodation available," and told us to go back to Bangalore and return the next morning and to keep doing this until they found some place for us to stay.

That was *how* we were introduced to the rural posting with no basic infrastructure or planning.

We did this for a week till some kind of makeshift accommodation was provided for us to stay. By the standards we were used to, it was a punishment, as the room was poorly furnished with no attached bath, and for our food, we had to rely on nearby hotels. A real introduction to rural life, we thought.

We sort of got used to this hardship and escaped to the city on weekends after spending five days learning rural medicine in that PHC [Primary Health Centre].

The ANM was a fat woman who had to walk a lot, often several kilometres. She did this with ease, and initially, we found it difficult to keep pace with her. She was a fun-loving person and regaled us with stories related to her job. She was the one who told us the secret behind the doctors at the PHC not wanting us to be around when they were busy seeing the patients.

The doctors were supposed to see the patients free, as the PHC was state-owned, but they collected a fee clandestinely and sometimes openly. As they provided a much-needed service, people had to come to accept their clandestine practice.

She had her own ways of working. We accompanied her when she went visiting villages. Her job involved keeping track of pregnant women, anyone who was ill, and those who were on long-term treatment for chronic diseases. This required her to visit several houses.

But she did nothing of that sort. She plonked herself in the village centre, either on the square built around the sacred peepal tree or at some house that had a verandah. Thus ready, she would open her ledger and call out to the passerby. It went like this:

"Ye, Range Gowda, has any woman delivered?"

Range Gowda would answer, "Yes, Thayamma, that lady Hanumi has, ten days back."

"What happened to that old man Sidde Gowda? Is he still alive?"

"Yes Thayamma, he is still alive." Thayamma would make appropriate entry and allow Range Gowda to take leave.

The next victim was Abdul Razak. His wife was pregnant.

Thayamma asked Razak in Kannada, "*Eno, nin hendthi hengide?* [How is your wife?]"

Razak replied, "Good."

Thayamma next asked, "Has Gowri visited her?"

You may wonder who this Gowri was. She was the village *dai* [midwife] who conducted most deliveries in the village, and

309

Thayamma kept track and registered the births in her register. She spent an hour or two doing this. She needed to visit one or two houses if there was a new patient or a woman who had become pregnant.

She took pride in introducing us to her admiring audience. She called us 'two doctor *ladke*' [two young doctors].

Many years later, I experienced how important this cog of ANM is in our healthcare delivery. I visited basic health services in rural Rajasthan a couple of years ago and saw how well the health centres can be run by trained local men and women, with periodic visits from the doctors.

The senior doctor gave us assignments as he pleased, as ours was the first batch, and there were no clear-cut instructions as to what and how he and his colleague should teach and train us. But he did spend some time talking about the various central and state government programmes that the health centre was implementing and the difficulties they were facing in doing so. Even though he indulged in collecting a fee, we found him well-informed and treated the mostly poor patients with courtesy and care. No wonder there was always a rush of patients at the centre.

We spent three weeks doing this domiciliary work, visiting the villages that the health centre served, and then we were seconded to a team of health workers headed by a social worker [sociology graduate]. This team was researching to find out which were the preferred methods of family planning.

Then, sixty years ago, the government was just waking up to the need for the nation to limit its numbers. There were four methods that were being tried. First was the use of condoms. The next was the pill. Third was the safe period, and the last was vasectomy. The team headed by the social worker visited homes and small businesses, with us tagging along. The team had already been working in the field for several months.

310

The first place we went to was a small shop whose owner had preferred condom use as his choice. He had requested the team to bring him a supply. So, the social worker proceeded to give him a packet.

The man asked her with some irritation, "What is this?"

The lady had to explain. "Last time we came, you had agreed to use this for limiting the family."

The man was now visibly angry. He said with a raised voice, "I do not need this; I never asked for this nonsense. I am not even married."

Then who was sitting here when we came last? Could it be his twin brother or his lookalike brother? It turned out to be his brother. We asked him where he [the brother] had gone?

"To the city," he said.

Obviously, he was reluctant to follow this method and thought it fit to avoid the team altogether. But he had failed to brief the brother. Matters of sex are dealt with a sense of shame and not to be shared even with your brother! The team was experienced in these matters and took it in its stride.

The next visit, after a few successful ones, was to a couple who were following the safe period method. This works in women whose menstrual periods are regular and whose ovulation days are accurately calculated. The first ten days and the last ten days are deemed safe to have sex. To help, the couple was given a frame with blue and red beads. What the man had to do was to move one bead a day, and on the day of the blue bead, the couple could have sex. It was taboo on days when it was a red bead day.

In a couple of homes, it was good news, and none had become pregnant. It was not so in the fifth home. The lady was visibly angry as she had become pregnant. As this was the least effective method, the team was not surprised. One curious team member asked the woman, "Did you follow the one-bead-a-day rule?" She replied, "I did, but my husband did not." The cat was out of the bag. The man, when he got the urge, moved the beads until the blue appeared and went ahead.

The next episode was with a woman who had agreed to follow the contraceptive pill method. This was popular and possibly the most successful of all methods tried. This lady, Kaveramma, appeared put-off by seeing us.

The social worker asked her, "Have you been taking the pills?"
"Yes, but it is of no use; I have missed my periods for three months."

"Are you taking the pill every day for three weeks and giving a gap of one week before starting the next cycle of three weeks?"

"Yes, I did. I took it for one week and did not for another week. I saved the tablets and gave them to my friend. Now she too is pregnant!"

This lady had heard the instructions wrong, and instead of three weeks on and one week off, she had made it one week on and one week off. This magnanimous lady has also donated the tablets to her friend and messed up with her cycles too!

Despite these infrequent mishaps, by and large, people were receptive to the idea of a small family. But they were reluctant to discuss matters related to sex in the open, and a lot of tact was needed to broach this subject in those days.

Our nurse Thayamma and that social worker were *experts*, and we learnt a lot about how to discuss this delicate subject from them.

❖❖◆❖

Dropping a Brick
(Written some years back)

There are numerous castes and sub-castes that divide us Indians. One such caste is the Brahmins. Among this large group, there are hundreds, if not thousands, of subgroups, and one of them is the predominantly Tulu [a dialect]-speaking Brahmins who reside in the coastal region of Karnataka.

As in any other caste, for the social functions of these communities, only those who belong to this sub-caste are invited. Therefore, when I found a *Tambram* [short for Tamil Brahmin], Thyagarajan, at one such function, I was naturally surprised. I knew Thyagarajan well and wondered if his wife was a Tulu Brahmin, thus qualifying him for the invitation by marriage. But I had met his wife, and she did not look or behave like a Tulu Brahmin woman.

Still, I was glad to see him after two years and went to him to exchange pleasantries. Seeing me, he gave a smile of recognition and asked how I was doing. I said I was fine and asked him, "Thyagu, how is it that you are here at this function?"

He appeared surprised and said, "My name is not Thyagu; it is Srikrishna, and Colonel Acharya is my father-in-law."

The function was a housewarming ceremony for the Colonel's new home, and naturally, the son-in-law had the right to be invited. A bit crestfallen at the mistaken identity, I apologised, and my apology was well-received.

Some months later, I met him again at another function, which was secular and included people from all communities, as the local bank had organised a customer meeting. This time, when I confronted him, I began, "You know, Thyagu, about what happened last time..." and proceeded to narrate the story of mistaken identity.

313

He heard the story in stoic silence and then said, "Doctor, I am sorry to disappoint you, but I am not Thyagu. My name is Srikrishna, and we met last time at my father-in-law's housewarming ceremony."

I was taken aback. Such an uncanny resemblance and similarity in speech! Again, apologies were in order but were accepted with some asperity.

There was another function where the participants were mostly Tulu-speaking Brahmins, and this time, too, I found Thyagarajan—*sorry, Srikrishna*. I made sure that he was indeed Srikrishna before going to speak with him, determined to get it right the third time.

On seeing me approach, he hurriedly got up and walked to another corner, obviously afraid that I would once more call him Thyagu!

I did not have the heart to chase him to prove to him that this time I had indeed made the recognition right.

❖❖❖❖

Backbencher

I am comfortable sitting at the back at any function, be it a continuing education meeting, a wedding reception, or a civic get-together. This habit I acquired some sixty years back in medical school. Then it allowed me to unobtrusively leave the hall through the large French windows placed strategically on the sides of the lecture hall. In those days, the lecturers took no offence if they noticed one's absence.

This habit has stood me in good stead and gives me ample opportunity to leave midway without offending the speaker or the organisers. On rare occasions, when I have to don the mantle of a speaker, I keep a subtle watch on the back rows to see if anyone is leaving midway, a sure sign of boredom/inattention. I am rather fortunate that it has not happened often.

In those bygone days, the continuing education programmes were simple affairs with a lunch or high tea thrown in at the beginning or the end. The speakers mostly depended on memory and experience and spoke extempore. Naturally, some of them bored us to death, and being a *backbencher* came in handy to take unobtrusive leave.

Has the advent of advanced audiovisual aids motivated me to occupy front seats? Sadly no. I find it has made matters worse. The modern-day speakers, with rare exceptions, have taken to reading these projected slides and not addressing the audience. A droning voice combined with dimmed lighting is conducive to sleep, and it is with difficulty that I keep my head up and eyes open. This goes unnoticed if you are a backbencher.

When I compare the speakers of yesteryear to the present ones, the ones of the past get a higher score. Maybe, being old myself, I am biased. I remember vividly my Neurology Professor, the late M.K. Mani, miming *grand mal* and *petite mal* [now the modern neurologists have named these differently] while speaking on epilepsy. Similarly, I remember another M.K. Mani [great teacher, alive and kicking] speaking on hypertension, though with the help of slides but hardly looking at them.

Lately, I have been facing a piquant situation. Thanks to my seniority and mop of grey hair, I am easily spotted and given our penchant for recognising [respecting?] old age, I am forcefully escorted to the front row of chairs, much to my discomfort. Here again, there is some hierarchical distinction. The frontmost row is generally a row of cushioned sofas or well-padded chairs meant for VIPs and thankfully the organisers have not recognised me as one, and they usually make me sit behind these.

315

The front-row occupants generally come late, and the importance is based on the position they hold rather than on any achievement, academic or otherwise. By arriving late, they also hold up the proceedings. In one such meeting, a serving police official of ill repute was the chief guest at a professional function. I felt happy that I was not in that front row, sitting with this worthy.

It is a different matter in social functions like weddings and receptions. Being the family doctor for generations of families, I often get invited to many of these, which even include ceremonies associated with death. Often, I have the *dubious distinction* of having presided over these deaths.

Readers should not get the impression that I am another Dr. Harold Shipman who killed many elderly. In my case, these patients were terminally ill and died under my care at home, and I saw to it that unnecessary hospitalisation and the resulting expenses were avoided.

Weddings, however, are joyous occasions. Normally I try and avoid these ostentatious and wasteful ceremonies. But sometimes I have to attend as the families concerned are too close for me not to.

Recently I went to a wedding. I have known the girl, a third-generation patient, since her birth. She is now based in the United States and the young man, her groom, is German. The girl's father and mother and the grandparents from both sides also were/are my patients. Both the grandfathers are dead [under my care at home], but the ailing grandmothers pushing eighty, are very much alive. So, this intimate relationship made it impossible to avoid this wedding.

The simple wedding ceremony was over, and the time arrived to bless the couple. Normally the elders of both sides take the first honour, followed by other relatives and friends. In this wedding, this tradition was broken, and I was ceremoniously escorted to the platform where the bride and groom sat and was requested to initiate the process.

It must have been a *spectacle* to the well-dressed gathering to see this *chappal*-clad, shirt-and-trouser-wearing, nondescript old person belonging to another caste and community being escorted to initiate the holy process.

This kind of affection, respect, and love makes us family physicians feel that we made the right choice in opting for this branch of medicine.

◆◆◆◆◆

When Nature Calls... From Above

Before we became independent, the British ruled us. There are many opinions as to the way they managed the affairs of the nation. But it is generally agreed that they did a fairly good job of administering this large country. This is especially true of the young officers who managed the districts and *talukas*.

These men were fresh out of their home country, and after the initial training, were posted to isolated places, thrown into a culture and people far removed from their own. Yet they managed to provide the best possible service to the population. They also wielded enormous powers over the subject population under their care. The following story is that of one such young officer:

He liked the country and the people and enjoyed the reputation for being fair and honest. He had to work hard to know his people, and to do this, he had to tour extensively. Some towns he could visit in his car, but often he had to go on horseback. He would start early in the morning after his breakfast and return in the evening. Often, he stayed on the outskirts of a large village in a specially designed tent.

There was one *blemish* that often ruined his otherwise healthy, fun and adventure-filled life. He suffered from constipation. Often, for days together, his bowels were bottled up. Help from the civil surgeon, who was a fellow white man, made matters worse. Consultation with local varieties of doctors of different disciplines, too, did not help.

Each morning, the young Sahib would wake up and wonder what was in store for him that day. If he had a bowel movement, his day was made; if not, he would remain grumpy till the next day and wait.

One such morning, after having failed to get his bowels to move, he gave up the attempt as it was getting late for his rounds. He had a hurried breakfast and left with his driver, attendant, and the office clerk who carried the relevant records about the villages the Sahib would visit. The attendant carried Sahib's lunch and other requirements.

The journey began. They must have gone a few miles when the Sahib started getting strong bowel contractions. This made him feel good. He asked his driver to stop the car at the nearest water body and urged him to hurry.

Soon they reached a bridge with a stream flowing underneath. Sahib got down and, having collected his all-purpose mug, hurried down to the bank of the stream. He undid his trousers and sat down for the much-awaited evacuation. *Alas!* The strong and urgent contractions disappeared as suddenly as they had appeared. This was no uncommon experience for the Sahib. He knew that if he waited long enough, he would get the contractions again, and his bowels would move. So, he sat patiently with his trousers down. But he kept his solar toupee on to guard against the sun.

He must have waited for ten minutes when he felt a soft thud on the toupee and a splash of gluey muck which splattered down. He looked up in time to see a native hurriedly

318

scampering down from his perch on the side wall of the bridge. Unmindful of the state he was in, the Sahib shouted, "Catch the *bugger*, don't let him go, I will come up and take care of him."

The witnesses to this awful spectacle—the attendant and the clerk who were sitting by the side of the car—ran and were able to stop the shivering native who by now had become aware of the enormity of his offence. He begged for mercy from the Sahib's assistants, who, by virtue of their proximity to the Sahib, were in themselves frightful figures.

By now, the Sahib, came panting up the slope without his toupee and shirt, which he had thrown into the stream and washed off the gluey muck as best as he could. He saw the poor villager being beaten by his attendants. He asked them to stop and went to the shaking, shivering, and thoroughly frightened villager who stood with folded hands, fear and despair writ large on his face.

No sooner had the Sahib came near him than, looking at this *half-naked white apparition*, the villager was overcome with intense fear, making him fall to the ground begging forgiveness.

Sahib asked him to get up and said, *"Hell with your apology,* just tell me how you managed to do the job so quickly."

The rest of the story is irrelevant.

❖❖❖❖

Lost in the Jewels

Among the many positive attributes of my friend, the late Gnandev Kamath, was his ability to tell a story. What follows is a real-life incident in which he was involved:

There was a wedding in the family and the relatives from far and wide had gathered. As it happens everywhere, weddings and deaths get the maximum number of relatives to come and meet each other. One is to celebrate a life-giving event, and the other to pay respects to a life which has departed. The former is a joyous occasion and thus much more attractive.

Gnandev's niece was one of them who had come from Bombay [now Mumbai] with her jewellery box to attend the wedding. The advice that she should not carry her jewellery and make do with borrowed pieces from her close relations was not heeded. Which self-respecting young woman likes to be seen in borrowed jewellery? My sympathies are all with her for bringing her jewellery with her at some risk.

Bombay is next door to us SKites [*South Kanarites, Mangalorians, Mangus, Coastal Cracks*]. There are hundreds of buses which ply daily from Bombay to Mangalore, and the flight connections from Bombay to Mangalore are better than those from Bangalore to Mangalore. The Bombay party, which included this young woman, duly arrived in Mangalore, and from there they travelled to Udupi, where the wedding was to take place.

The day before the wedding is the day of fun, where women have the maximum opportunity to display their person, and if that is not worth it, then at least their jewellery. As our young lady in question had both, one can understand her anxiety to be ready for the evening function. She stayed in her relative's house, and at the appointed time she travelled to the venue.

When she reached the venue, she found that her jewellery box, handbag and her mobile phone were all missing. She had forgotten the whole lot in the auto-rickshaw in which she had travelled!

All hell broke loose, and the lady was inconsolable. The reasons were many: the lost opportunity, loss of jewellery worth many lakhs, and the ignominy of being branded as a forgetful woman for the rest of her life! All these and many more added to her grief. The promise of the gathered relatives that they would all contribute and make good her lost jewellery was not well-received.

The only option was to go to the police. She, of course, did not remember the auto's number and could vaguely describe the driver.

Before going to the police, why not try the mobile phone that she had left behind in the auto, and maybe the driver would respond? Normally, the first act of a thief is to remove the SIM card and throw it away. When they rang the number, there was a ringing tone, and this reassured them to some extent. Continued tries, however did not elicit any response, and they were now worried that the mobile phone's battery would die, and then they would be in deeper trouble.

At this moment, a thought occurred to Gnandev. He requested the assembly to close their eyes and pray silently for five minutes, wishing for the recovery. Five minutes elapsed, and Gnandev made a final call to the mobile number before going to the police.

The phone rang only twice before it was picked up. The voice at the other end said that the jewellery box, handbag, and mobile phone were with him and he would return these to the owner. It would take him some time as he was 30 kilometres away. It took some convincing to get him to stay home and wait for Gnandev to go there and collect the lost and found articles.

When Gnandev reached the driver's place, he found it to be in a poor locality, and the anxious driver was waiting to give it all back. They found that he belonged to a goldsmith's community and knew the exact value of the jewellery in the box. Not a single piece was missing. He was wondering how to reach the owner when he heard the mobile phone ring!

When they wanted to publicise his honesty, he would have *none of that*. It took a lot of pressure to persuade him to accept a cash gift.

It was pretty late when they went back to the venue where the evening's party was on. The thanksgiving revelry went on till the wee hours of the next day.

It is because a few of these men and women [first class of humans] are still present in this country that we are surviving.

✦✦✦✦

Lovers of Noise and Sound

We Indians, irrespective of community, caste, or religion, celebrate our festivals, rituals, our worshiping of many gods and goddesses, and our music festivals with a lot of noise and sound. Loudspeakers are a *must* in most of these functions. The louder the sound, the better the fun.

If it is for a few minutes, though disturbing, as it happens with the piercing call for prayers from the nearby Masjid or a loud announcement by the passing BBMP garbage truck preceded by loud music, one can put up with it. But if the noise and sound are an everyday affair going on for months together, it becomes a headache and annoyance to the likes of yours truly.

Throughout the city are spread what are known as Ayyappa Swamy *bhakta mandalis*. These are groups of devotees of a deity called *Swamy* [saint] *Ayyappa*. Ayyappa is a Kerala-based deity with a massive following in South India, spread across all Hindu communities. This crazy [my take] following results in a yearly pilgrimage to Sabarimala [where the shrine is located].

Before the devotees leave for the venue, they gather at these places of worship and pray for several months. These prayers begin at 7 pm and can go on to midnight, depending on the fervour and stamina of the gathering.

One such group existed near me. If the prayers were subtle and the sound did not carry to kilometres around, I would not have minded. But the loud, repetitive prayers [*noise* for me] for days and months, daily in the evening, were disturbing, to say the least. There are laid-down rules for loudspeaker use, and the rules are generally flouted, as was the case here.

I sent word to one of the devotees whom I knew and told him about my discomfort. He said, "No one else is complaining except you." He assured me that they would tone down the loudspeakers. But this did not happen.

I had no option but to lodge a police complaint, which I did. The police wanted a written complaint naming the perpetrators. I did not know the members but wrote 'Ayyappa Swamy bhakta mandali, Marappan palya' as the perpetrators of this auditory crime.

What happened next was hilarious when I look back.

Sundaran Pillay is a long-time resident of Marappan palya. At the time this incident occurred, some thirty years back, he had just retired from HAL [Hindustan Aeronautics Limited] and had taken it as his life's mission to propagate Ayyappa Swamy. This I came to know only later.

He and his family of wife, a daughter and three sons were then in various stages of settling down, and all of them were my regular patients. Keralites make good patients in that they are educated, understand what you are saying, follow advice, and return for follow-up on the appointed date; they are also good paymasters. Sundaran Pillay and his family were no exception to this.

So, when he came to see me apparently healthy, I was a bit surprised. I asked him, "How are you? And what is the problem?"

He was quiet for a while, wondering where and how to begin. At last, he said with an aggrieved tone, "The Police have stopped our prayers for two days, and I came to know that you had lodged a complaint."

"I did not ask them to stop your prayers; I only asked them to see that you all follow the rules on the use of loudspeakers," I said. I also reminded him of my request sent through Krishnan, a fellow devotee, and a friend of his.

"But they have removed the loudspeakers and taken them away and warned us to dismantle the deity's platform," he said.

I had to agree this was police excess.

"Now what should I do?" I asked him.

He said, "You please withdraw your complaint, and I will assure you that we will tone down the sound."

I agreed and went to the police station the next day. The conversation with the Sub-Inspector [SI] went on like this:

The SI started saying, "Doctor, we have confiscated their sound system and told them to stop the illegal activity; if they don't, I will file a disturbing public peace case against them."

This was too much, and my intention was not to stop the activity but just to reduce the noise. I explained this and told him that my complaint was only to get them to follow the rules regarding loudspeaker use.

"Do not worry, Doctor; they cannot use them. I brought the sound equipment with me," the SI said.

It took some more pleading for him to understand what I was saying. Then somewhat sobered down, he asked me to write another letter withdrawing the complaint, which I promptly did.

I was about to leave when he called me back and said, "If you are going that way, take this sound equipment and loudspeakers and give it to them."

This, I thought, must be *Swamy Ayyappa's doing*—that I, the complainant, had to carry the offending equipment and hand it over to Pillay and the other followers.

It might be of interest to know that his sons are well-settled, as is the daughter. Two grandsons are in the United States. All of them remain my patients, though they and their families live in different parts of the city.

Pillay died of prostate cancer many years back. His wife, too, died some five years back, peacefully at home, following my advice to her eldest son not to hospitalise her.

❖❖◆❖

In Search of Applause
(Written some years back)

Someone held a spoon with a lemon on with his teeth for 47 hours and 55 seconds and has entered the Guinness Book of Records, said the daily. That this "mad feller" went through the ordeal just to get into a record book by doing this weird act is a fact that doesn't surprise me, because I see several such acts committed by people around me. This craving is almost universal among humans and is likely inherent in our psyche.

If one cannot achieve this recognition by one's own merit, then one will buy it; this seems to be the modern Indian credo. Some examples:

Kishendas Bikamchand is my patient and friend of many years. Bikam, as he is popularly called, is a very successful businessman. He belongs to a community whose members are well-known for their business acumen, and many of them have dominated the commercial scene of the country, and one can even see them on the world stage [Laxmi Mittal, for one].

One day, Bikam came to my clinic with his daughter's wedding invitation in hand. He said, after the preliminaries, that I must attend the wedding, which was taking place in faraway Jaipur. He extended the invitation to my wife also.

Seeing the obvious reluctance on my face, he said, "Doctor, you don't worry; I will take care of the money that you are going to lose by not practising for three days. I will also buy both of you business class tickets and fly you back." He was serious when he said this. I had to decline the invitation despite the incentives he offered.

Bikam met with me after the gala wedding. I asked him how much he spent on the wedding. He said, 'Rs. 5,00,00,000 [Five crore]'. The floral decorations alone cost him Rs. 5,00,000 [Five lakh]! Even Rajasthan government ministers attended the wedding, he said *proudly*. When I said what a colossal waste of money, he replied that unless he did that, how would his community know he had succeeded, and how else would his daughter get the respect from her husband's family?

"So, when your son gets married, will you expect the prospective girl's parents to spend an equal amount?" I asked.

"No, more; because the cost will be more, as one has to keep pace with inflation!"

Bikamchand is not a bad man. On the contrary, he is a very good, fun-loving, helpful person, but the illness of craving for recognition from his community drove him to this *irrational act* [for me, that is].

M.R. Reddy is a small-time contractor and politician in this locality. With some difficulty, he became a member of a local club. Every year, the club holds elections and elects a committee to manage the affairs of the club. The elected members are given various responsibilities. One gets to run the kitchen, another the sports section, and yet another the bar, and the like. These members, in turn, form what are called subcommittees consisting of their cronies to help them.

M.R. Reddy's friend, who got elected, got the bar section of the club to run. M.R. worked overtime to influence his friend to get him on the subcommittee. Once he was on the subcommittee, he went around telling everyone he knew about this tremendous achievement. I was one of the recipients of this information, and my congratulations were warmly received.

A month later, I got an ornate invitation card kept inside an equally ornate envelope. This was the invitation for the marriage of M.R. Reddy's sister's daughter. The envelope, in one corner, had this legend: "With compliments from: Mr. M.R. Reddy, Member, Bar Subcommittee, HAL Club!" Needless to say, I did not know the groom's nor the bride's parents. Reddy took it upon himself to invite the two thousand-odd members of the club to his niece's wedding!

I came across a letterhead of a gentleman who went one step further. The top of the page had his name, and among equally mundane accomplishments was that he was an ex-member of the City Club!

But there are some who want to achieve not for fame but for the sake of a purpose. You can place sports persons, adventurers, and social workers in this class. They do the job for the pleasure of it, and if they also get the recognition, so be it.

There are, of course, some who deserve to be recognised but go about doing their job without bothering about recognition [the late Dr. K.T. Achaya, T.N.A Perumal].

❖❖◆❖

Story of a Sri Lankan Guide
(Some facts and some fiction)

We, a group of golfers with our wives, went on a golfing and sightseeing tour to Sri Lanka some fifteen years back, and we had an interesting guide named Santo. I don't know why he chose me for comfort and advice. It all began like this.

"Sir, I hope you don't mind me asking you," he said.

"Certainly not," I said.

"Sir, I don't know why Mr. R doesn't like me." I asked him how he knew this.

"Yes, I know. I heard him say that I take a cut from the shops I take you people to," he replied.

I asked him, "Santo, have you ever worked as a cook?"

This question took him by surprise. He must have been wondering what a cook has to do with the problem he has come to discuss with me. He said no, he had no experience as a cook.

"Suppose you worked in a kitchen as a cook, will you not taste the food?" I asked.

Now he brightened up a bit and said, "Yes Sir, I will. Otherwise, how I know the food is good?"

I explained, "The same thing is true with tour guides. They must taste the items they make the tourists buy." Now he was visibly happy.

328

"Sir, you really think so?"

I said "Yes." But still, he lingered. "But Sir, he thinks I take money."

I told him it did not matter which *form* one tasted it in.

"Sir, I cannot do it; I am a Buddhist," he replied.

I said, "Buddhist or not, you are a guide, and you must first taste the food before you make us eat it."

He left saying, "Thank you, Sir, for your advice."

Another day he came to the room and said, "Sir, I have one more problem."

I asked, "What is it now?"

"Sir, that old man [all of us were old, but he singled out one], Mr. P, asks difficult questions."

I said, "We tourists don't know which questions are difficult and which are not."

"But Sir, it is not once but many times, and today he asked me why Buddhists do not follow family planning. I told him, 'Sir, there is no state policy,' but he said the state does not say when one must have sex; it is an individual's decision; you are a Buddhist; you should know."

"Sir, how can I answer this question?"

I said, "You be quiet and don't answer such questions."

"Sir, I did, but he will not leave me. 'Santo,' he tells me, 'Why are you quiet? You did not answer my question.'"

"So, what did you tell him?" I asked.

"Sir, I told him I don't know about Hindus, but we Buddhists enjoy sex."

I came to like Santo. I asked him what Mr. P said to that.

"Sir, he became quiet, but I see he is not happy with the answer."

I told him I was very happy with the answer. Santo appeared pleased with my response.

"But Sir, I cannot upset people."

I told him, "Don't worry. Mr. P will be secretly happy; old men of our age just talk about sex whereas you guys are still in the game." A very pleased Santo left me.

Another day and time.

"Sir, another problem; Mrs. K thinks that the store where we went this morning sells fake jewellery."

I told him, "All costume jewellery is fake."

"Why Sir, you too think so?" I said that the jewellery being sold was not made of silver or gold; it was all plated.

"*Aaah*, that kind of fake, that everyone knows."

"But Mrs. K doesn't," I told him. "She must have heard that in Sri Lanka jewellery is cheap, and she must have been disappointed to find it is cheap because it is plated," I added.

"I will be careful hereafter and tell all Indian women tourists that the jewellery is plated; they will not blame me for taking them to a fake store," Santo said before leaving.

A day later, another problem.

"Sir, that man who always has a serious face." He found it difficult to remember the name. I told him he is Mr. S.

"Yes, Mr. S; he says why is it raining here always? You should provide umbrellas to all."

"Sir," he continued, "Do I make rain?" I said, "No."

"That too not in season?" For this also I replied in the negative.

"Then why, Sir, this gentleman wants an umbrella at all times?"

I told him, "See, Santo, why do some people always wear a coat, even when it is hot?"

He said he did not know.

"That is because it is a habit. Mr. S carries an umbrella all the time when he is in Bangalore, and that is why he wants you to provide an umbrella, and because he cares for others, he has included all of us."

"But Sir, giving umbrella to all twenty-one is difficult, but still I will tell the company for the future [he made a note in his diary]."

From the umbrella, he jumped to another topic.

He said, "Sir, I am also a sportsman."

I became interested and wondered why he was telling me this. I asked him what sport he played. He said, "I play billiards."

I said, "Very good." [felt the game suits his paunch]

"Sir, do you play billiards?" I said "No."

"Sir, billiard is also like golf; you put the ball in the hole, but area of play is small, not like golf." He waited for my reaction.

I said, "Yes Santo, but golf is easy."

"No Sir, golf very difficult. In golf you have to walk all over, get wet in the rain, hit a small ball with a long stick, get leg pain; then Sir, you must *drink beer* after you finish."

I agreed with most of what he said but not the last part. I told him, "Drinking beer is not compulsory. We drank beer because Sri Lankan beer is very good."

He beamed with this appreciation of Sri Lankan beer.

"But Sir, there is one gentleman, Mr. P, who drinks only Sri Lankan arrack, not good for his age; you are a doctor; you tell him not to drink like that."

I told him, "Santo, that Mr. P can drink a bottle of arrack and still play a round of golf."

"OK, then Sir don't tell him; let him drink Sri Lankan arrack; only two days left [for the tour to finish], you know."

Another day.

"Mr. S, he don't like me."

"Why not, I saw him with you, talking and laughing this afternoon," I said.

"Talking yes, but no laughing, no Sir."

"Why does he not like you?" I asked.

"Not liking, not in that sense Sir; he does not like me sitting with you yesterday at dinner table. I think he belongs to superior caste. In India, I think you have this caste—superior and inferior. I have heard."

"Santo," I said, "You are a Buddhist; you belong to the most superior caste, and you have the right to sit at the centre of any table."

"Sir, then why he told me so?" Santo asked.

"See, Santo, that Mr. S, he is a big businessman; he wants to talk business, and if you sit with him, he cannot talk business but only about the tour; that is why he told you not to sit at the table."

This placated him. "Oho so; but I will be careful [another note in his diary]."

"Sir, Janak thinks you all are very good people."

This unasked-for compliment from the bus driver took me by surprise.

I asked him how he had classified us thus.

He said, "All of you wish him before getting on the bus."

If being good was *just wishing*, then the whole world would have been of good people. I kept quiet.

"But there is one person, Mr. S, who has not wished him so far," Santo complained.

332

I asked him, "Why are you telling me this?"

He said, "I tell for your future reference." What it meant I do not know.

On the day of leaving Santo came to see me one last time. He said, "Sir, this tour was very good; you all are such good, educated people." "Your wives *also*," he added as an afterthought.

I asked him, "But you had so many complaints?"

He said, "Sir, that is for my education. Last tour group had only Germans; I suffered so much I cannot tell you; your group very good."

On that salutary note, our Sri Lankan golf-cum-sightseeing tour ended.

(The tourist guide's dialogue is presented verbatim, to maintain authenticity.)

❖❖◆❖❖

A Glass of Water

This article, a real-life experience narrated by plastic surgeon Dr. Neha Chauhan, appeared in the *Indian Journal of Cancer*, and its editor, Dr. Sanjay Pai, has permitted its publication in this book, along with my comments.

*****

Cancer management is developing at a rapid pace. Since it requires a multidisciplinary approach, in most large cities dedicated cancer care institutes have come up that provide holistic care to cancer patients. Most cancer patients directly approach these centres for specialized care. Plastic surgeons play an important role in reconstruction following excision of malignancies but owing to the reason stated above, it is rare for a freelance plastic surgeon, not working at a cancer institute, to encounter such patients. And rarer to write about such an encounter!

This is a (real) story of my rendezvous with Mr. SN. My first meeting with Mr. SN can't be described as a pleasant one, not even in the wildest of imaginations!

Before I begin my narrative, I wish to briefly outline the facility that led to my brush with Mr. SN. The general surgeons at our hospital have an attached dressing room while all the surgical super-specialties share a common dressing room. I being a plastic surgeon dealing with trauma, burns, and reconstructions, occupy this other dressing room (henceforth referred to as dressing room 2 or DR2) for a maximum duration of time on any given day. Almost all my patients need dressings and going by the teachings of my MCH [an advanced post-graduate program in surgery] professors, I never (I repeat never ever!!) hand them over to anyone else. I have hence, been declared the uncrowned queen of this DR2 by the staff who time and again joke that the DR2 should be officially declared as the Plastic Surgery headquarters for all practical purposes. Being the one who has kind of usurped the DR2 ever since I joined, I have always enjoyed the privilege of finishing my dressings first.

All was going as per the routine until one fine day when my queendom stood challenged! And the one who challenged was none other than Mr. SN! He had been shifted into the dressing room by the staff on instructions of the spine surgeon and for one whole hour, he occupied the DR2 as the surgeon had not yet finished his OPD consultations and was not able to come to the room to dress him. The patient could not be moved in and out of the room again and again as he was paraplegic and recently operated on. Hence, the staff gave me a sorry look and asked me to wait until the spine surgeon came and finished the dressing. Left with no option, I returned to my OPD room and finished evaluating my remaining patients.

By the time I came back to the dressing room, another hour had passed by. However, to my dismay, the spine surgeon had not yet arrived and my patients had started breathing down my neck complaining that they had been waiting for nearly two hours for dressing. Although I could empathize with SN's condition, somewhere inside I was fuming (in all probability due to the challenge posed to my territory). Added to this, nagging by my patients and their attendants raised my temper further. With great difficulty, I swallowed my anger and decided to wait until a call from the OT sister broke the last straw of my patience.

I had posted a case at 2 pm but some emergency case had come up which they wanted to post at 2 pm. Since the OT was free before that they wanted me to start my case at 1 pm and finish it before 2 pm or else to operate only after 7 pm. A quick glance at my watch and I realised that it was already 12:30 pm and all my patients requiring dressings were still waiting for DR2 to be vacated. With all my patience tested, I marched towards the staff nurse seething with anger, and expressed great displeasure at their lack of coordination with the doctor. I suggested that next time they should take any patient inside only when the concerned doctor had come to DR2 and not in advance and thus block the room causing inconvenience to other patients for hours at a stretch. She responded by saying that she was just a staff nurse and could not say no to orders from any doctor.

Mr. SN and his attendants were all ears to this conversation and by the look on their faces, they were not exactly pleased by my suggestions to the staff nurse. To my relief as soon as my conversation with her ended, the spine surgeon arrived. He finished dressing, SN was shifted out, and I hurriedly finished my dressings and headed to the OT. This was my first meeting with SN!

I had learnt from the staff nurse that SN would come for dressings on alternate days and I made it a point to finish my dressings before he came so that I never encountered him but little did I know that fate had different plans! I kept bumping into him or his attendants almost every other day for the next couple of weeks, somewhere in the waiting area or near the dressing room. Needless to say, the look on their faces suggested that there was a kind of cold war going on at my supposedly unconcerned and unkind suggestions to the sister at SN's first visit.

Over a couple of weeks after my first brush with him, I learnt that SN had been operated on for some spinal tumour. A month into my first encounter with Mr. SN, I had almost forgotten the incident when the spine surgeon called me one evening asking me if I could see one of his patients who had developed wound dehiscence following surgery. I asked him to send the patient the next day to my consultation room. To my surprise, the patient was none other than SN! He and his attendants were aghast to see me. With great reluctance they let me see Mr. SN's wound. He was having marginal necrosis with total dehiscence of the surgical site and frank CSF leak. He looked much weaker and exhausted than when I had seen him for the first time. He coughed badly and was diagnosed as having severe bronchopneumonia and uncontrolled diabetes besides the wound problems.

On going through his medical history, I came to know that he was eighty-three years old diabetic, operated on for a spinal tumour at the level of the 9th thoracic spine a month ago. He and his family at the time of diagnosis itself had made the decision that they would let the spine surgeon remove the tumour in the hope that the patient's paraplegia improved but in case it turned out to be a malignant tumour they would not want any adjuvant therapy. Histopathology and immunohistochemistry had revealed it to be a low-grade B cell lymphoma but the patient only wanted palliative treatment.

It was decided that the patient would be admitted under the spine surgeon for observation of CSF leak besides being treated for bronchopneumonia and I would look after his wound and daily dressings. After discussion with the patient, it was planned that once Mr. SN's pneumonia improved, the CSF leak would be repaired and flap cover would be done for his exposed spine so that the quality of his remaining life would not be compromised.

Nervousness was palpable on both sides! From their looks and attitude, it appeared that the patient party was not very comfortable with me managing their patient. On the other hand, even I was not exactly keen to manage a patient whose family did not trust me or my intentions. After a long deliberation and convincing by the spine surgeon, the patient agreed to be treated by me. For the first 2 days, I would visit the patient daily, do his dressing, write my notes, and come back. I wanted to talk to the patient but he was too breathless to talk. Attempts to talk to the attendants were also not paying off as they were reticent for the initial two days.

336

On my third visit, the patient's general condition had improved a bit. As soon as I wished him good afternoon and he opened his mouth to respond, I noted his dry tongue. A glance at his urobag showed dark-coloured urine. The next question was a spontaneous, "Are you thirsty? Would you like to have some water?" Back came the response in affirmation with a nod of his head. The attendants had been asked to wait outside till I finished my dressing and the sister had gone to arrange for a dressing trolley. So, I spontaneously picked up the glass kept on the table beside his bed and poured water from a bottle kept there. SN eagerly snatched the glass from me like a child and in a matter of seconds drank the entire glass and asked for one more. I happily obliged.

I was all smiles inside somewhere patting myself, at having diagnosed his dehydration when he broke the silence and said "How did you know that I wanted water? You will become a very good doctor one day. You can read through a patient's mind. I was thirsty for quite some time now and wanted to drink water but doctors and sisters have been coming for rounds back-to-back and then they had started me on nebulization so I could not drink water." I finished my dressing and went to write my notes, after which I left the hospital. This was my first conversation with SN! And it left me happier as that awkward silence was broken.

On my fourth visit, he had improved a bit further clinically and to my surprise opened up to me about his family, life, and profession. His family also shared with me the challenges they had been facing since he was diagnosed with a tumour. They told me how his life came crashing down one fine day when he suddenly developed paraplegia. According to his family, he was an extremely self-reliant person his whole life and the news of the tumour had broken him completely inside. On my next visit, he had a childlike excitement in his eyes and told me that his childhood friend and his wife were coming from Chennai to see him. He excitedly shared what he had asked his wife to cook for his childhood friend and how he had been asking his son to call her every now and then to know if everything that his friend liked was on the menu.

Over the next four days, I gained the trust of the patient and his family and they would share important events of the previous day with me. They had become comfortable with me and I had renewed enthusiasm to treat the patient who showed trust in me. After all, finally, they and I were on the same page that they would let me try my best to heal his wound. Rest they wanted to leave to God.

Suddenly, SN became critical the next day and needed ventilatory support but he and his family had decided against the same when he was fully oriented and had signed a note in advance at the time of his admission. To my disappointment, by the time I reached the ward they had already left with him against the advice of his primary doctor and I could not meet SN that day. As I was leaving, the staff nurse handed me a note they had left for me. I opened it with trembling hands. It said, "Thank you doctor for all your efforts but he wants to spend his last days at home. Hence, we are taking him."

I do not know how long he would survive but 'the glass of water' that broke the ice between him and me is going to stay in my memory for quite some time. On reflection, I realised how a small spontaneous act, as small as offering a glass of water, changed my equation with the patient. A patient party that had been almost at war with me (sans the visible weapons of destruction!) had suddenly started respecting and trusting me and my treatment. I realised that there may be times when we may not have an exact solution that can cure patients but small acts of kindness that show that we care for them can ease their pain a bit and help them spend their last days well. This is especially true of patients with cancers. Even with all advancements and pathbreaking research, we will many times encounter situations where we cannot scientifically help such patients much.

As I walked to the DR2 with a heavy heart, Leo Buscaglia's quote echoed in my mind, "Too often we underestimate the power of a touch, a smile, a kind word, a listening ear, an honest compliment, or the smallest act of caring, all of which have the potential to turn a life around." This incident brought to my mind the famous quote by William Osler that I could not comprehend when I read it for the first time as an MBBS second-year student.

As I reflect, I also wonder at what would have been my response had I drunk a 'glass of water' myself when I was fuming on the very first day of my encounter with SN. Could it have extinguished my anger resulting in a calmer approach to the staff, no cold war from the patient party, and lesser stress to myself? Well... that only a 'glass of water' would be able to answer, when I drink it next time I am displeased with a situation beyond my control!

Till that happens, I leave the readers to reflect on the Hippocratic advice of "Cure sometimes, treat often, and comfort always!" This quote perfectly sums up what we, as crusaders of cancer, need to remind ourselves at all times.

*****

Henceforth, these are my own comments, as per the editor's request:

Below are three quotes I have taken from this real-life experience shared by Dr. Neha Chauhan.

• "You will become a good doctor *someday*."

• "*Cure sometimes, treat often, and comfort always!*"

• "*A good physician treats the disease; a great physician treats the patient who has the disease.*"

Most of us become good doctors as we progress in our profession if we have the right attitude. The very sick Mr. SN realised that Dr. Neha was, after all, not a bad doctor when he was given that much-needed glass of water. He did not say, "You are a great doctor," but instead he said, "You will become one *someday*."

When we enter medical school, many of us harbour high ideals of service and compassion, along with similar aspirations to help the sick and needy. During the many years of gruelling training, these ideals often take a back seat. They

339

are replaced by ambitions to achieve status, earn money, and climb the social and professional ladder.

Patients and their ailments become steps in this direction. In the bargain, many of us ignore health, sleep, exercise, family, friends, and other interests. Real happiness becomes a casualty, and quality of life suffers in this pursuit.

Focusing on disease management often takes precedence over treating the patient as a *whole person*. This is especially true as doctors specialise. When one is stressed with work, especially the work as described by the doctor who is a plastic surgeon working in a cancer hospital, where he or she must be seeing many seriously ill patients, one is in danger of becoming inured to suffering.

One major complaint many patients have is that we are not concerned about them. One hears patients stating, "He did not even place the stethoscope on my chest," or "He did not even ask me why I am there," or "He just looked at my reports and wrote out a prescription." Often, we take our patients for granted and do not think that their concerns are of great importance, as we already know what is wrong and what to do.

However, patients have many worries and anxieties and want to share these with us. We must listen to them, even if they do not always make sense to us.

We sometimes forget that our patients are often highly accomplished in their own fields, and they are here as patients *not by choice but out of necessity*. When we seek help from other professionals, say an engineer or an accountant, don't we expect courteous interaction? We, more than in any other profession, need to be better at human relationships because we are dealing with suffering.

If one removes the relationship between us and our patients, we become mechanical robots, often very efficient ones, as many of us must have become. This is the death knell of our profession. Whether brief or long-term, the doctor-patient relationship is *essential* for the satisfaction of both.

As aptly described by Dr. Neha, the act of giving a glass of water triggered the development of this relationship and made her progress towards becoming a good doctor.

This relationship is not just with the patient but also with the patient's family, relatives, and other well-wishers. It is not merely medical but also social and psychological. Can one have a relationship without getting affected? The answer is *no*. Involving oneself in the social and psychological aspects of a patients' illness can be distressing. However, one needs to participate and be a part of patients' worries and concerns, and not infrequently, their joys.

We, more than in any other profession, have this unique opportunity to become better human beings if we learn to treat patients as *persons* and not as collections of organs.

There is also a possibility of us being healed as well!

❖❖❖❖❖

Mind and Medicine

When we look at a flower, we know in an instant that it is a flower. We also know what type, what colour, and what smell it has. We also know how, where, and when to grow that plant. All these different qualities of the object 'flower' are possible to perceive because of the highly specialised brain cells located in the cerebral cortex. When last mapped, there were thirty such areas to interpret visual imagery *alone!*

Think of our sense of smell, taste and sound and the various interpretations that we do with these sensory inputs. So too is thought and its association in our brains. The latter quality has led to what we are today and has enabled the human mind to construct and also to destroy.

But the last word has not been said about the brain. There is a huge uncharted territory out there to explore. I recommend to those of you who want to know more, to read books by Vilayanur Ramachandran [*The Emerging Mind, Phantoms in the Brain*].

Norman Cousins died in 1990. His life and work made me think and approach human health and disease from an angle that is *different* from that of the taught clinical approach of fitting the known symptoms and signs into a known disease. Keeping the human being as the centre and then looking at his or her problems gives one a different idea of the nature of suffering, and often one can solve the problems where conventional wisdom has failed.

In my early days of practice, it would frequently surprise me, but now it no longer does, as I am becoming more and more aware of the enormous healing power of the human brain.

Norman Cousins wrote several hugely popular books [*Anatomy of an Illness, The Healing Heart*]. The lives of the likes of Cousins and Ramachandran are fascinating because they have, within the confines of our present-day knowledge, tried to explain the disease phenomena and suggest *unconventional* cures.

What we know today about ourselves is only a fraction of what we do not know. That is why Norman Cousins called today's medicine *Frontier Science*.

❖❖✦❖❖

True to the Oath

The 1st of July is celebrated in India as *Doctors' Day*. Every Doctors' Day, I get a bit overwhelmed to receive so many calls and SMS messages from my patients. It is in the fitness of things that I remember a few doctors who really lived up to the oath they took to serve the people.

The earliest was my own general practitioner, Dr. Shanbhag. My memories of this doctor go back to over sixty years. I was a very sick child, prone to many respiratory illnesses. It was a rural setting in which Dr. Shanbhag practised. His wife was his assistant. He handled all ailments, and I remember an episode when I was unwell with whooping cough, and he sat with me when I was racked with paroxysms of coughing. He was overworked, poorly paid by his patients [they could not afford it], took no precautions to remain fit, and died in his fifties of a heart attack.

It is surprising that I encountered no one truly memorable during my medical school days. However, one person who deserves to be remembered is Dr. Sarosh Patel, about whom I have written previously. There were a few seniors and colleagues who lived up to the *Hippocratic Oath*; they too died prematurely.

The first of these was Dr. Manjappa Gowda, who came from a farming background and remained a simple farmer at heart until a fatal heart attack claimed his life. Unlike others, Dr. Manjappa served as a general surgeon in the government health service. His skills under adverse working conditions were legendary. He was known to act as both anaesthetist and surgeon, and with the help of assistants he had trained, he performed all kinds of surgeries, often under spinal anaesthesia. This he did in settings with primitive facilities— in rural and semi-urban areas. His personal life was full of tragedies, which he bore with great equanimity. His solace was tobacco, which probably contributed to his early death.

Next is Dr. M.R.R. Rao, who was unfortunate enough to have been born with polycystic kidneys, which ultimately took his life, though he had some extension because of a successful renal transplant. He was one of the first to return to India, spurning offers of a very lucrative career in the United States thirty-five years ago. He was way ahead of his times and was brilliant in everything he did. He pioneered the use of endoscopes and attempted arterial grafts. Many of us who had our patients operated on by him remember his skill and commitment.

The last to pass away was Dr. Malathi Rao. A specialist surgeon and a gynaecologist, she also returned to India, giving up a very promising career in the United States. She too like Dr. M.R.R. Rao was a pioneer. She trained scores of doctors in the use of laparoscopes. She was also the first to introduce endoscopic uterine procedures in Bangalore. Latterly, she was doing excellent work in the field of infertility. Sadly, she succumbed to cancer after a courageous battle with the disease.

There are a few others who are alive and practising true to the oath they have taken, but I am reluctant to write about them because they are still living. But the large majority, for various reasons, are not committed to their oath, and this is not the occasion to write the why and what of it.

There is one thing that was common in the lives of all the doctors whom I have written here. They placed the interests of the patient above other considerations and were prepared to pay a price. None of them made a lot of money, though they could have, and none went after recognition or status.

They lived up to their own set of high standards and were *worthy examples* for others.

✧✧◆✧

344

10

FACE TO FACE WITH EMINENCE

Vijay Raghavan Thiruvady

Mr. Vijay Raghavan Thiruvady had been my patient and friend for over fifteen years. That we had common interests strengthened the bond between us. He had multiple health problems, and these needed constant care and surveillance. That he lived eighty-two years, a full life, with many serious health problems is in itself a lesson for others.

He died suddenly of a heart attack some time back, leaving a legion of nature lovers grieving. Vijay was justifiably famous for his encyclopaedic knowledge regarding the trees of the subcontinent, especially those one sees in the urban setting such as in the city of Bangalore. His weekly walks in Lalbagh, taking a group of enthusiasts, were a *must* for nature lovers who lived in the city and those who visited from outside.

While writing one of my articles, when I was at a loss to identify a set of trees that I had come across and sought his help, I was rewarded not only with the name of the tree [*Kauri Pine*] but also its ancestry and the associated legend.

He was also a historian and based his talks on well-researched facts. His walks in the Lalbagh and Cubbon Park gardens and the sprawling campus of the MEG [Madras Engineer Group] centre were like history books of the past three hundred years of the city opened in front of you.

345

Adding to the knowledge, a flair for storytelling and keeping himself in the background made Vijay *unique*.

His death is an irreparable loss.

❖❖◆❖❖

Dr. Subashchandra
Subash, as I knew him.

It was some thirty-five-odd years back that I went to Chennai [then called Madras] to visit a patient of mine who had undergone a coronary artery bypass graft at the Madras Mission Hospital. It was there that I first met Subash, who had just returned from the United States and was looking after my patient post-op [post-operative care]. Incidentally, this patient is still alive and healthy.

What began as a casual acquaintance then grew into a friendship that became closer and closer as the years went by and remained so, until his untimely demise.

There were many reasons for this strong bond. We shared many interests other than medicine, such as birdwatching, literature, old books, and music, to name a few. We also came to know ourselves as individuals with shared values. Subash, being a person of *impeccable integrity*, was often at loggerheads with the corporate hierarchy, and on occasion, this was the topic of our discussion and how to manage some of these tricky situations that he would often get into.

His dedication to work, the kind of cardiology practice he had built up, and his ability to get along with people helped him overcome the many problems he faced in his illustrious career. He was a great interventional cardiologist and a selfless team leader.

Being older [not necessarily wiser], I was privileged to be privy to his confidences on more than one occasion, and I

346

fondly recall the time we spent discussing issues related to and sometimes unrelated to medicine and the ethical dilemmas we often faced.

Over these three and a half decades, I have referred patients with cardiac problems ranging from acute MI [Myocardial Infarction] to sick sinus syndrome, various types of heart block, tricky septal defects, discordant ventricles, and the like. On many occasions, he has managed my patients who would have otherwise died.

He is also responsible for helping me to interpret TMT [Treadmill Testing] tracings when I was unsure of the advice given to patients that it was positive and further investigations like angiography and stenting might be required. Quite often, his advice that the test results were normal saved my patients a lot of trouble, unnecessary hospitalisation and related expenses. There were several other occasions when his advice greatly benefitted my patients.

I cannot count the number of instances when I have disturbed him in emergencies, often at night, and the response was always the same—quick and to the point. Many beneficiaries of his professional expertise and experience are today alive to tell the tale of their recovery.

Some years back, while culling old books in my club's library, I came across a 1904 edition of Sir William Osler's book *Aequanimitas*. Knowing that he collected old books, I presented it to him, and I am sure it occupies a prime place in his library.

For nearly thirty years I ran an organisation called the Family Physicians' Association [FPA], primarily to educate and update doctors, and Subash was a regular teacher whenever a cardiology topic was being discussed.

For the past thirty years, I also run a small group of fifteen doctors called the Doctors Club. We meet once a month mainly to update and discuss difficult problems that we have faced or are facing, and here, too, Subash was a valued invitee.

Let me conclude that all lives are precious, but *some more than others*, and my friend Subash's was one such.

I miss him.

❖❖◆❖

S.S. Acharya [Shagari Srinivas Acharya]

It was in the year 1969 that I first met Mr. Acharya. I was scouting around to find a suitable place to begin my practice. This area [the present-day Indiranagar] was just beginning to develop but was mostly rural, and Mr. Acharya was among the first to settle here after his retirement.

Most of his service was in Calcutta [now Kolkata], and his family spoke more Bengali than their native tongue, Tulu [a dialect]. My uncle had asked me to meet up with him to get the hang of the area as a potential location for my starting practice.

Thus, one fine afternoon I landed at his place and rang the doorbell. It took a while for the front door to open, revealing a dour elderly gentleman dressed in khaki shorts and a white banyan. Later, I realised that this was his standard mode of dress for all seasons. He was unhappy, as it was probably his siesta time and to have been abruptly woken up.

I made a quick introduction and dropped my uncle's name. At this, his demeanour changed, and a smile appeared on his face, and he welcomed me into the house. He made me sit on a hard chair and made himself comfortable on an easy chair. Many years later, he told me that it was his ploy to make unwanted visitors uncomfortable so that they would leave early. But then he also told me that some visitors had no shame and sat for hours despite the discomfort.

348

Mr. Acharya, after having seated me on that uncomfortable metal chair and coming to know the reason for my visit, proceeded to grill me as to my origin and antecedents. Normally, such personal queries end up annoying me, but then here I was, a visitor, welcome or not, and had to respond to his questions.

At last, after this test, he seemed to be satisfied with my pedigree and proceeded to give me a talk on what he expected from a doctor, frequently quoting the example of his family doctor in Calcutta and telling me that I too should be like him—to be available at all hours, never to lose cool, and to keep service as the primary objective in life, *etc.*

The interview lasted more than an hour, and after being satisfied that I was a good listener, he gave me a cup of tea and wished me good luck. Thus began our fifteen-year relationship, which lasted until his death some thirty years ago.

Mr. Acharya was a diabetic and insulin-dependent. Tragically, he was also very fond of food. Though I became his trusted doctor, I don't think I succeeded in adequately controlling his diabetes.

Being from the same area and belonging to the same clan, we would often be invited to the same social functions. Mr. Acharya would wait and watch where I would be before he took a seat, as far away from me as possible so that he could eat his meal in peace, away from my watchful eyes. He took an extra dose of insulin before committing these 'crimes'!

Mr. Acharya owned a nondescript car that he was very fond of and maintained it himself. Often, I would find him with greasy hands tinkering with the innards of that car. Once I even found him spreadeagled under the car with his scrawny legs sticking out! He would make trips to Shivajinagar *raddi* shops in search of spare parts for his car. Though this car was a liability [my opinion], Mr. Acharya did not think so and turned a deaf ear to his wife's entreaties to buy a new car!

He was also fond of gardening and had flower bushes and fruit trees in his backyard, and on many occasions, he would bring a fruit or two or some flowers and present these to me with pride and pleasure. As my consulting place was close to his house, it was easy for him to take a walk and see me.

He had a trying time during his last couple of years. He developed a complete heart block and suffered a stroke. In those days, this city did not have any cardiac intervention worth the name. As he suffered frequent episodes of syncope [losing consciousness briefly], he needed a pacemaker. This was available in Manipal. Mr. Acharya went and got this done, and though his syncopal attacks ended, and his quality of life was better in a way, his hemiplegia troubled him and put an end to many of his interests.

For me, it was painful to see him going around with a stick and a lopsided hemiplegic gait. He suffered another stroke and lapsed into a coma. I withdrew all the medications, and he passed away a week later at home.

Even now, when I pass by the road where his house once stood [the present-day Chinmaya Mission Hospital Road], these memories come flooding back.

✦✦✦✦

Dr. [Capt.] Thimmappaiah

It was sometime during 1972/73 that I first met Dr. [Capt.] T and remained his friend till he died some fifteen years ago at the ripe old age of ninety-two.

Those were the days when, compared to now, communication was primitive, and the only options were either to meet in person or use the telephone, which only a few lucky ones possessed. There was a three-year waiting list for acquiring this valued instrument, though, on paper, doctors were supposed to get it out of turn!

Having found myself out of date as far as medical knowledge went, I was looking for avenues to update myself, and the only active body was the local IMA [Indian Medical Association] branch, located in the heart of the city. I tried calling to find out if there were any ongoing programmes, only to find *staccato noise* at the other end!

I decided to pay a visit to the IMA house. IMA house, then and even now, houses the state and the local city branch under the same roof, and I went there one afternoon. Considering the time then, the building was impressive, and the city office was located on the ground floor. A few tables and a couple of chairs with filing cabinets furnished the office. Most were empty except one, which was occupied by an elderly gentleman who, I later came to know, was the manager and ran the office and the office bearers.

I made my enquiries as to the CME [Continuing Medical Education] programmes. While I was talking with him, Dr. T made his entry.

Dr. T was always impeccably dressed in a dark-coloured suit, and with his tall and slim frame, he cut an impressive figure. Added to this, his fame as a cricketer, athlete, social worker, and ex-army officer helped to enhance this aura. At that time, I did not know all these additional attainments of his, but from his demeanour, I could gather that he was a doctor. I introduced myself, and after he learnt of my army background, he became very friendly, and the next half-hour was spent telling me about his own army experience on the Burma front during the Second World War. There was not a hint of bragging in narrating his exploits.

I think he must have decided that I was worthy of being in his inner circle at that very first meeting. He then proceeded to tell me about the various activities of the IMA and how it needed to improve its academic programmes and invited me to be part of them.

During the next couple of years, I became the secretary of the IMA College of General Practitioners of the state, and my friend Dr. S.K. Srinivasan the state secretary. We began running a series of educational programmes, which sadly ended a couple of years later as the state and the local units were taken over by doctors who had little interest in academic activities. We were forced to start our own association, which came to be known as the Family Physicians' Association [FPA], which has grown to be a body of nearly a thousand members now.

Let me get back to Dr. T. During his school and college days, Dr. T was an athlete and a stage artist. Being good-looking, he was given female roles. This necessitated shaving his arms and forearms, as you cannot have a hirsute man playing a female role.

On one occasion, after the performance the previous evening, there was an athletic meet the next morning where he was taking part in the 200-metre run. The athletes duly took their stance, and next to Dr. T was Abdul Khaliq, a classmate and fellow competitor. Khaliq told him, "Thimmu, what is this? All the hair on your arms gone? I thought you only shaved the beard area; have you now begun this new fashion of shaving your arms also?" This was to distract Dr.

T. Irritated, T replied, "*E thuruka* [slang for Muslim], you concentrate on running and not on my shaven arms!"

Dr. T was a more than average cricketer and played for Karnataka in the Ranji Trophy matches and has the distinction of being the first one to score a century for Karnataka in a Ranji match. He was also a medium-pace bowler, and when he was in his mid-fifties, was seen bowling to Dilip Vengsarkar, some thirty years his junior. More than a player, Dr. T was known as a cricket administrator. He, along with Mr. Chinnaswamy, was instrumental in building the present stadium, which goes by the latter's name. After the demise of Chinnaswamy, Dr. T became the President of KSCA and remained at the helm for several years.

He was active in the affairs of the IMA, and I remember on one occasion going with him to attend a national conference at Lucknow. There were five of us, and I have vivid memories of that trip. One of us was in chronic cardiac failure and had poor effort tolerance but insisted on doing what others did, and being the youngest, I was put in charge of this doctor. As he was on diuretic tablets, he needed to urinate often, and finding a loo/convenient spot was a major problem. He would often [jokingly] threaten me with this imminence. Throughout the three-day trip to and the three-day trip back, I remember playing poker with no loss of money.

Another vivid memory of Dr. T on that trip was his stopping play when we approached Whitefield station on the journey back and going to the lavatory. When the train was approaching Bangalore East Station, he emerged, clean-shaven, with his trademark suit on.

The West Indies and Indian Test teams were being hosted by him as the President of KSCA, and he was getting down at Cantonment station and had asked his nephew to come to the station to ferry him to The West End Hotel, which was close by. Ten minutes later, he bade goodbye to all of us and made his regal departure.

The present IMA building came up because of Dr. T and his friends, to name a few: Dr. Subramanyam, Dr. Nagaraj, Dr. Ashwathnarayan, Dr. Shivram, and Dr. Ramaswamy. I may have missed some names. All these stalwarts are no longer with us.

He was also interested in classical music and started his lessons when he was in his mid-thirties. A lady teacher would come home to teach him. Dr. Subramanyam would often pull Dr. T's leg, saying, "Our Timmu's wife also began learning, not because of any interest in music but to keep a watchful eye on the music teacher"—may not be without substance, given Dr. T being so handsome.

As I know, he was the president of a co-operative society, a bank, a music association, and the Indian Red Cross.

One is justified in wondering how he managed his clinic located in the city centre on Kilari Road. I once asked him. He said, "When I get time, I go there and open the doors. Patients come to know that I have come, and they arrive, and when they are finished, I close the doors and go. I earn enough to keep my body and soul together."

This was Dr. T!

Though very fit, his last years were plagued by backaches and sciatica, which he bore with a lot of grace.

✦✦◆✦

354

Dr. K.T. Achaya

The December 22, 2008, issue of *India Today*, under the caption "Currying Flavour," carried a review of a book titled *The Illustrated Foods of India*, written by Dr. K.T. Achaya. The reviewer, I felt, did not do justice to the personality of the late Dr. Achaya.

Dr. K.T. Achaya was a remarkable person in more ways than one. By training, he was a chemical engineer who branched out to become one of the foremost authorities on oilseeds. So much so that he published several monographs on how ancient Indians extracted and processed oil from oilseeds. He had to consult several books, visit many temples, and study Pali and Sanskrit, and he did most of this *after his retirement.*

He was a serious student of Indian cuisine and made an in-depth study of how foods are preserved and prepared in different parts of the country [*Your Food and You*, National Book Trust, India]. His *A Historical Dictionary of India* [Oxford India Paperbacks] is a must-read for anyone interested in the origin and migration of many items of food that we take for granted.

To give a few examples—the chilli that you are very fond of is not indigenous but was brought to India, probably by the Portuguese, from South America. And the popular potato has the same origin.

The Story of Our Food [Universities Press] is a fascinating account of various Indian foods and how they came to be cooked the way they are cooked now, the different utensils that were in use to prepare the foods, and how these evolved.

His *Everyday Indian Foods* [National Book Trust, India] is a storehouse of definition, preparation, processing, and storing of popular foods from different parts of the country. So much for his talent as a food technologist, writer, and researcher on Indian foods.

Now let me come to some other aspects of Dr. Achaya. He was a connoisseur of classical music, both Indian and Western, and had a collection of records that he would lovingly play on his old record player. His knowledge of musicians and their lives would hold me fascinated.

He was also a very knowledgeable amateur botanist and could name the plant if you took a pod, a flower, or a branch of a tree. When I was with him, a lady from Kerala visited him with a round green fruit and wanted to know what it was. Achaya spent the next ten minutes telling her about the fruit, its uses, where it is grown, and the whole works.

He was also an art lover, and original paintings by many famous artists hung on the walls of his flat.

This man from Coorg never lived there. He spent the early part of his life in Madras [now Chennai] and later lived abroad, and after his return, he lived in Bombay [now Mumbai] and Hyderabad.

He settled in Bangalore with his sister and brother-in-law. His brother-in-law was a famous Lieutenant-General [I have forgotten the name]. His sister, Sitha, was a famous doctor, and before her retirement, she was the Principal of Lady Hardinge Medical College, Delhi. It was some twenty-five years ago that I met him initially as his doctor and later became his friend.

Dr. Achaya remained a bachelor. He was dogged by diabetes and heart disease, both of which he bore with rare equanimity. It was a privilege for me to be associated with him and look after him in the last years of his life.

❖❖◆❖

Dr. Vainu Bappu

I am writing about Dr. Vainu Bappu, forty years after he passed away. His life spanned only fifty-four years, but in this short time, his achievements were many.

These came about at a time when India was under the stronghold of politicians and bureaucrats who were brainwashed into socialistic thinking and acting. Scientific innovations and the building of institutions like the Indian Institute of Astrophysics [IIA] and the observatories that he built and nurtured were *not at all easy*.

This shows what kind of man and leader he was. Many honours came his way, including that of *Padma Bhushan*, and he bore all this with humility and simplicity. That he was a man of such achievements was known only to his professional colleagues and others like me who were close. The rest came to know only after reading the citations [these can be accessed on the internet] from his colleagues like Dr. J.C. Bhattacharya, who succeeded him as the director, and Prof. Radhakrishnan.

Here I confine myself to what I know of him as a gentleman who, in addition to being a great astronomer, was also an extraordinary, multi-talented human being. The years I spent looking after him, from 1973 to his death in 1982, were a privilege.

It was a call from his friend and my patient, Mr. Nedungadi, that led to my first meeting with the Bappu couple. Both Vainu Bappu and his wife, Yamuna, were staying in Hotel Brindavan off M. G. Road when Yamuna developed a severe bout of vomiting and dizziness, and I was asked to do a house call. That was in 1973, when Dr. Bappu was busy with the construction of the Indian Institute of Astrophysics in Koramangala. I went and visited them in the hotel room. Yamuna was in bed and very scared, as the dizziness was

357

severe. Moving her head to the right would bring on an attack of severe giddiness.

This condition is called Benign Paroxysmal Positional Vertigo [BPPV]. Usually, we doctors give some name which the patient will not understand, and, in this case, we must have failed to find one such name and thus given this condition such a name. In ordinary English, this means Benign [not serious], Paroxysmal [coming in waves], Positional [related to head position], Vertigo [intense giddiness]. *So much for the name!* In the next three days, she became normal enough to move about and fully recovered in a week.

They moved to their house in Koramangala, and I became a regular visitor there. Later, they used to come to my clinic in Indiranagar. Our friendship blossomed and did not end with Vainu Bappu's untimely death, as his widow, Yamuna, continued to be my patient for the next thirty years, and, at the time of writing, she is alive and keeping reasonably good health.

Dr. Bappu and I shared several hobbies—a love of cricket, books [he, like me, was a Wodehouse fan], music [he had a collection of classical music records], nature [he was an authority on roses], and a love of trees. The garden around the Indian Institute of Astrophysics is full of exotic rose bushes, and once he took me around and explained the pedigree of each bush. He also loved trees, especially those that bore profuse flowers like *Cassias* and *Tabebuias*.

In the seventies and eighties, the treatment for heart disease, compared to present-day standards, was primitive. If my memory serves me right, Dr. Bappu began developing symptoms some four or five years before his death. The ECGs suggested a compromised blood supply even while resting. Interventional cardiology was unknown in India, and even in the United States and Europe it was still in the developing stage.

If the present-day facilities and expertise were available then, I am sure he would have had another ten or more years of quality life. It was not to be, and when he was in Munich to participate in the conference of astronomers as the President of the International Astronomical Union, he suffered an acute episode, and the surgical procedure to revive him failed.

He left behind thousands of his admirers grief-stricken. He was only fifty-four years old, and he packed such a lot of achievements into this short span of life.

When he found out that his ECGs were not normal, he began studying the electrophysiology of a normal heart and what happens when the blood/nerve supply gets compromised. He would get into a healthy discussion on this subject. I used to marvel at his grasp of the subject, and I needed to read up to answer some of his queries.

I still feel a sense of loss whenever I think of him which is often. Vainu Bappu was one extraordinary human being that I have had the privilege of being associated with.

A link to his biography and achievements, authored by one of his colleagues, is provided below.

https://www.ias.ac.in/article/fulltext/joaa/003/03/0217-0218

❖❖◆❖

Shanbhag and his Bookshop

Premier Bookshop, located on Church Street off M.G. Road [Mahatma Gandhi Road], closed operations a few years ago. With this, an era of selling books came to an end.

Forty years back, in the early years of my general medical practice, I made little money and had lots of time. I spent this time reading. The only places where books were available cheap were a lending library located some distance away and second-hand bookshops off M.G. Road and Balepet. The bookshops that sold new books were many, but the one that drew my attention was Premier.

I would first visit the second-hand bookshops and then go over to Premier. The books I took home were generally second-hand [used] and thus cheap. Even these purchases were few and far between. But I liked the look and feel of new books and loved reading them. So, I frequented Premier.

Unlike other bookstores in that area, Mr. Shanbhag of Premier was a book lover himself, and he and I soon discovered each other *for what we were*.

This is how it happened. I would go and stand there in front of the rows of bookshelves, select a book, and start reading. Time would go by, and I would shift from one leg to the other. After some time, I would stop and then go home with my used books, either borrowed [from the lending library] or bought from some other shop.

On one such occasion, seeing me shifting from one leg to the other, Mr. Shanbhag came to me with a stool and requested me to sit and read. Thus, I could continue for an hour from where I had left off on the previous visit. But this was not an ideal arrangement, and his bookshop was not meant for itinerant, impoverished book lovers like me. However, the man's heart [or business sense] was large.

Another day, while I was busy reading, he came and said, "Would you like to take it home and read?" *Wouldn't I?* As long as I brought the book back in the same condition that I took it in, it was OK with him. This relationship between us, which began with no profit to the owner, blossomed, and I began buying books when I could afford them.

I have written elsewhere about the part I played in starting and nurturing the Indiranagar Club. When I became a committee member, I was given the responsibility of buying books for the club's library. This was the moment to repay

Mr. Shanbhag for all the consideration he had shown me in the past. During my time overseeing the club's library, I bought books from him.

I continued to visit his bookshop for many years until access to M.G. Road and parking there became difficult, at which point my visits became less frequent. But of the many persons who have shaped my character and life, Mr. Shanbhag, the bookseller and book lover, must take a *prominent place.*

❖❖◆❖❖

Roger Binny

Roger Michael Humphrey Binny now holds the exalted position of President of the Board of Control for Cricket in India [BCCI]. According to some, this post is equivalent to that of a Chief Minister of a state, in terms of money and power. That these sit *very lightly* on the broad shoulders of Roger Binny can be seen by the demeanour with which he conducts himself whenever there is an occasion where he is supposed to head the proceedings.

More often than not, he delegates this to Jay Shah, the BCCI's secretary. That the latter enjoys the limelight is another matter. Some say that Jay Shah manages to be around on such occasions, and Roger doesn't. Knowing Roger, this is believable.

Though I have known him for over twenty-five years, initially as a friend and later more intimately as his doctor, I only became even closer to him later, when he took up playing golf, as we would often play together.

I first met him under strange circumstances. In the late eighties, he built a house and settled with his family in my neighbourhood. The aura of the 1983 and the 1985 wins, where he had played a significant part, was still fresh, and his face was familiar to most of us. There was one shop that went by the name of *Videowala* in the shopping area of the neighbourhood, and this shop was popular as it hired out videos, the principal home entertainment in those days. This Videowala lent the videos to members only, and for non-members to become members, a member had to introduce them.

Thus, it came about that once when I was there, I found Roger looking for someone to introduce him. Though that was my first personal meeting with Roger, I had no hesitation in introducing him as a trustworthy person to this merchant. Thus began a friendship that only grew over the years.

Some aspects of this endearing personality are worth writing about. Foremost among the many is his self-effacing attitude. One has to push him for others to know him. Many honors and positions came his way, and all these came un-sought and un-canvassed.

He was the coach for the Under-18 cricket team, Chairman of the selection committee, President of the Karnataka State Cricket Association, and now is the President of the national body. All these positions he held and is still holding with *little or no fanfare.*

He has friends across the world, and some of us are privileged to know him not just as a great cricketer but as a simple human being who cares for others, including animals and plants. His love for dogs is legendary.

Once, while driving back home, he witnessed an accident where a mangled dog lay on the side of the road. Roger picked him up, took him to his vet, got the surgery done, and rehabilitated this half-lame dog at his farm. On another occasion, my wife found him leaning over our kitchen sink and gently rescuing a baby lizard with a spoon. This kind of love for animals may be the reason why he gave up eating meat some years ago.

362

He has a farm near Bandipur nature reserve where he is supposed to grow fruit trees like mango, pomelo, coconut, and the like. He has partially succeeded, and I don't think he makes any money from his farming activities, as wild elephants quite often raid his farm, despite the fencing, and eat the plants. He keeps losing his ripe crops, but does he blame the elephants? On the contrary, he says that he is the one to be blamed as it is *their* land he has occupied!

He has built a water tank next to his fence for the wild animals and has strategically placed a CCTV camera to capture the animals drinking, and I am privileged to see these videos. While elephants, wild hogs, leopards, and porcupines are common visitors, a tiger is an occasional visitor. There was one video where a porcupine was not allowing a family of leopards to come near the tank. They had to wait until he moved away.

There was another instance of elephants emptying the whole tank, leaving no water for other animals. This sighting of wild animals visiting is common in summer as the sanctuary suffers from water shortage. Despite the fencing, Roger has lost a couple of dogs to the leopards, and again, he is quite philosophical and even admires the stealth and accuracy with which these leopards do their hunting.

Outside his farm, it is mostly wild bush. It is leopard country, and sighting leopards is very common. While out on his morning walks, he has had many close encounters [sightings] with this wild cat.

Some years ago, there was a python that visited his farm, and Roger videoed its stay at the farm. Snakes of all varieties are regular visitors, and Roger has become, over the years, an expert snake catcher, and when he retires from the BCCI President's job, he can easily take up this job.

Roger spends most of his time on his farm, and he stays here in the city only when necessary. He now lives in a flat at

Kasturi Nagar near one of the metro stations, and during his time as the President of the State Cricket Board, one often found him walking from his flat to the metro station, getting into the metro, getting off at the M.G. Road station, and walking up to his office at the Chinnaswamy Stadium.

I wonder what he does now as the BCCI President. I would not be surprised if he takes a suburban train to the BCCI office from the airport!

Lately, since his becoming the BCCI chief, our meetings have become less frequent, and some of us close friends are looking forward to 2025, when he retires and becomes available to us to spend some quality hours playing golf and enjoying time at the *19th hole.*

❖❖◆❖❖

Gundappa Vishwanath

Another cricketing personality I am privileged to know and admire is Gundappa Ranganath Vishwanath, popularly known as G.R. During the decades of the seventies and eighties, when he played his brand of batsmanship, I do not think there was another player who was as admired as him. Like Roger, Gundappa also came from a humble background.

While the streets around Fraser Town and Cleveland Town were Roger's haunts, Basavangudi and Vishveshvarapuram in South Bangalore were Gundappa's. Graduating from tennis ball cricket to red-ball cricket and from school cricket to league cricket was not easy, especially given his middle-class, non-sporting background. How this came about is best described by him in his delightful autobiography, *Wrist Assured.*

Those were the days when West Indian cricket dominated the world. The names of Weekes, Walcott, Worrell, Sobers, and later Lloyd, Kallicharan, and Richards in batting, and W. Hall,

Gilchrist, Holder, Marshall, Roberts, Holding, and Garner in fast bowling were justifiably famous. In those days batsmen played without the protection of helmets. Vishwanath played most of his active cricket as a Test batsman against these fast-bowling stalwarts. Add the Australian fast bowlers Dennis Lillee and Jeff Thomson, and the list becomes even more impressive. I have left out the Pakistani and English bowlers lest the list become too long.

That Vishwanath's 6,000-odd Test runs came facing some of these fast bowlers when they were at their *fiery best*, and playing without a protective helmet, speaks of the little man's courage and ability.

When I say 'little man', I am speaking the truth. A more apt word to describe him would be 'little *great* man'. Little because he stood only 5 feet 3 inches in his boots, great because of his performance on the field and his behaviour off the field. Let me share two examples of his performance on the field.

It was in the 1979 Chennai Test against the mighty West Indies, who were then the best cricketing side. On a pacer-friendly wicket, India was reeling at 5 wickets down for 70-odd runs and staring at a possible defeat, with Vishwanath holding at one end. He went on to score 97 with the help of the tailenders, with a mix of impeccable defence combined with timely aggression, and this innings goes down as one of the greatest innings ever played by an Indian batsman. That he did not get his century was rather unfortunate.

As the cover drive raced towards the boundary, Vishwanath, thinking the shot would certainly get him the required four runs and the century, was ambling across, little realising that the ball had been fielded inside the boundary and the throw to the wicketkeeper had him well outside the crease.

While walking back, he had to listen to the curses in Kannada from the tailender B.S. Chandrashekar for not watching the ball, getting out, and depriving himself of a well-deserved century. Century or not, this innings of 97 has gone down in memory as one of the best, and even *Wisden*, the chronicle of cricket, has named this as one of the greatest innings ever played.

The other equally famous incident involved Vishwanath, this time as captain of the team against the English Test team, in what came to be called the Golden Jubilee Test played at the Wankhede Stadium in 1980. The Indian team had made 242 runs and had the English side reeling at 85 for 5 when this famous act of great sportsmanship occurred. Bob Taylor was batting, and Kapil Dev was bowling when the ball sped past the bat without touching the edge. But the umpire gave the batsman out, caught behind.

Although the umpire gave the batsman out, Vishwanath, who had been fielding at slip, consulted the wicketkeeper and called the batsman back after he had already begun a slow, unprotesting walk. Taylor and Ian Botham went on to score 171 runs, and England won the match. No one remembers the English win, but every cricket lover remembers the *exemplary sportsmanship* exhibited by Vishwanath on that memorable day.

He is a fun-loving guy and very easy to converse with. I came to know him only after he began playing golf some fifteen years ago. When, in one of the post-game sit-downs, he was asked how come he specialised in square and late cuts, he replied, "This was only against the West Indian fast bowlers, because by the time I sighted the ball, it was already at wicket level, and the only option was to cut the ball square or late; there was no chance of hitting it in front of the wicket."

The other story attributed to him was how he escaped injuries when facing fast bowlers in those years playing without a helmet: "No danger; I am only 5'3"; the balls hurled at me went easily over my head," he replied.

Both statements were made in jest and may not be factually true. But that is what Vishwanath is and a person to be with.

His biography, *Wrist Assured*, is a must-buy for all cricket lovers. It is a thoroughly enjoyable read.

❖❖◆❖❖

11
INFLUENCERS

Sardar Khushwant Singh

Sardar Khushwant Singh passed away in March 2014. I am one of his *unabashed* admirers and have been so for many years. What endeared me to him was the celebrated spat he had with that egocentric, difficult-to-suffer Krishna Menon, who was then Indian High Commissioner in the UK. I had then, and even now, a gut dislike for Krishna Menon and his acerbic ways of speech and behaviour.

To our then-naive Prime Minister, Jawaharlal Nehru, Krishna Menon could do no wrong. History now reveals that Krishna Menon was an *unmitigated disaster* as far as this country is concerned. His tenure as Defence Minister saw us suffer humiliation at the hands of the Chinese in the 1962 war. He, like Nehru, had a coterie of sycophants, and one of them was General Kaul, who had no idea of what was happening to our soldiers who were facing the Chinese. Krishna Menon gave the order to *throw the Chinese out*, which ended in utter rout of our ill-prepared and ill-equipped army.

Some old-timers will remember his tenure as our representative in the UN [United Nations] and his marathon verbal battles with Sir Zafarullah Khan and later with Zulfikar Ali Bhutto of Pakistan on the question of Kashmir. Krishna Menon would put even the most ardent admirers of his debating skills to sleep, and when they were not his admirers, like the other members of the UN, one can imagine how ineffective he must have been in putting our case across.

Very few had the .guts to take on this powerful man, and Khushwant Singh was one of them. He held the important post of Press Attaché and had to deal with this man day in and day out. On one such frustrating occasion [I have read the juicy details in some book], he seems to have thrown the papers at him and quit the post!

For many years, Khushwant was the editor of the magazine *Illustrated Weekly of India*. During this period, he saw the weekly's circulation soar by adopting methods that annoyed many purists but delighted the readers. Gossip with rancour, interspersed with a liberal dose of exposed female sexuality, was his *recipe* for success. Even later in life, he made no bones about his liking for wine and women and bemoaned his old age because he could no longer enjoy these.

In his long career as a newspaperman, he hobnobbed with the rich, the influential, and the famous but never became anyone's lackey. One can with some justification accuse him, in hindsight, of being close to the late Sanjay Gandhi. I remember a picture showing him at the wheel of the prototype of the Maruti car, which was Sanjay's brainchild.

Sanjay Gandhi had clear ideas which appealed to many of us. He was not taken in by the then-popular ideology of socialistic secularism. He believed that the country's escape from poverty depended upon compulsory family planning, afforestation, slum removal and beautification, and private enterprise. This has been proved right in later years, but the way he went about doing it was *draconian*, and large sections of the population went against him and his mother, as the election results then showed. But Sardar Khushwant defended Sanjay even when it was not the *popular thing* to do so.

One would, by reading the above lines, say that he was a *crass* person. Far from it. He was well-read and a learned person who had delved deeply into the history of the Sikh religion and wrote books on this. Though steeped in religion, he was an agnostic and did not believe in the existence of a formed God. His newspaper columns frequently lampooned godmen and godwomen.

Lastly, his humour. In addition to being a *ready wit*, he was also a collector of funny anecdotes and published these in a book. From one of these, I share below a witty story:

Santa Singh and Banta Singh ran an engineering contracting company. When the British and the French floated tenders for the tunnel construction under the British Channel, the lowest quotation was from this Santa and Banta firm, located in Jalandhar. It was so ridiculously low that they were about to dismiss it altogether as impossible.

But the tender rules did not permit this, and the brothers were duly called to appear before the committee. The brothers appeared dressed in their new suits.

They were asked, "How can you do it this cheap?"

"*Simple*," they said. "I, Santa, will dig from this end, and he, Banta, will dig from the other end. We meet at the centre, and there you have your tunnel."

Taken aback by this simple logic, they were queried further, "Mr. Santa, it needs great engineering skills and very expensive equipment to meet at the exact place; what will happen if you both miss?"

Santa laughed and said, "Why you worry? You get *two tunnels at the cost of one.*"

That was Sardar Khushwant Singh!

❖◆◆❖

Sir Garfield Sobers

Garry Sobers, as he was popularly known, played international cricket representing the West Indies for a period of twenty years, from 1954 to 1974. He was probably the most *naturally gifted* cricketer ever to have played the game. He didn't coach players to play the game by the rules; players to whom the game comes naturally do it differently, and Sir Garry is one of them.

Many rate Sir Donald Bradman and our own Sachin Tendulkar among the best who have played cricket, but my choice goes to this West Indian from the island of Barbados as the greatest of them all.

Do I have reasons to rate him higher than the other two? *Yes, many.* Sobers is ambidextrous, though he preferred to bowl and bat left-handed, as it gave him a natural advantage. He scored 365 runs in one Test match, a record which stood for many years. He bowled leg-spin, off-spin, medium-pace, and fast. He could also swing the ball very late. He excelled as a fielder, both close-in and in the outfield. They said he could also keep wicket!

Those who were fortunate to watch him in action said that they had never seen the likes of him. He was a five-in-one all-rounder and enjoyed himself *as only a West Indian could.*

There are many stories attributed to Sobers. One of them was that he spent a whole night partying, and one did not expect him to be on the field the next morning. To everyone's surprise, he was there on the field, *cold sober!*

West Indian cricketers are exciting to watch. They seem to have the ability to transmit their joy to the viewers. They play their cricket like no others do. Very few of them like to defend. For them, the ball is bowled at them to be hit. Hit they do, and in the bargain, many times they get out cheaply.

Despite this trait, they have produced some all-time greats, one of them being Brian Lara.

In 1974, the West Indian team visited Bangalore, and the present Chinnaswamy Stadium was under construction, and the stands were made of bamboo! I remember one shot vividly. I don't remember who the fast bowler was, but the batsman was Alvin Kallicharan. He went down on his knee and hook-pulled the ball out of the stadium. They were like that. They made shots that were not seen before.

Sobers once hit six sixes in an over in a first-class match, which was done again many years later by our own Ravi Shastri and more recently by Yuvraj Singh. Remember that Sobers played his cricket in the *pre-helmet* days!

Sir Garry took to serious golf after he quit cricket. Like many ex-cricketers, including our own Kapil Dev and Roger Binny, he, too, excelled in the game. Being ambidextrous, he played both right- and left-handed. His handicap during his best days was *1 left-handed* and *2 right-handed!*

Sobers is now eighty-eight, lives in his home country, and takes an active interest in promoting cricket in the West Indies.

◆◆◆◆◆

Bismillah and his Shehnai

Since I gave up my evening clinic work, I have found some idle time at my disposal. I use it for playing golf and badminton, afternoon naps, reading, and, more importantly, listening to music. Readers of my blogs are familiar with my love for Hindustani Classical Music.

Though my first love remains vocal music, I often listen to this music played on the *shehnai*. The shehnai is a reed instrument, and the note produced is smooth and easy-flowing. I find a lot of mental peace listening to the shehnai.

Common knowledge is that the instrument came to India along with the invading Muslim armies around the 10th century. I, too, was under the same impression until I read a well-researched article ["Indian Oboe Re-examined," published in the *Journal of Asian Studies*] written by Dr. Dileep Karanth [who, incidentally, is my wife's nephew]. Dileep is, by profession, a physicist and has other interests, as one can make out by reading this article.

Shehnai, in one form or another, has existed in old India since prehistory. It spread from there to other parts of the world, and the music played, of course, came under a lot of foreign influence, notably Sufi Islam.

The greatest exponent of the shehnai was the late Bismillah Khan. Bismillah died at the ripe old age of ninety in 2006. Honours came to him aplenty, including the *Bharat Ratna*. Despite all this, he remained a simple man, managing his large family and dependants. His home was the temple town of Benaras, and in one of the interviews, he said he found the presence of God while playing the shehnai on the banks of the River Ganga, which flows by Benaras. He often performed inside the Kashi Vishwanath temple.

In fifty years, he transformed the shehnai from an instrument played primarily during festivals and marriages into a principal instrument of Hindustani Classical Music. It is now performed on stage like any other classical instrument.

Though he is no longer with us, I have vivid memories of him playing the shehnai. It was a visual and auditory treat. I remember his face with the trimmed white beard and the laugh lines around his twinkling eyes. With a black coat and a white cap, he had a stage presence rarely seen these days.

What I liked about his music is that he rarely gave in to musical calisthenics to impress the audience. His music was smooth and easy on the ears and played as much for us as for himself.

Traditional music, as we have seen, is slowly disappearing. Shorter versions with more titillation seem to be the order of the day. But old music, like old wine, is still available thanks to quality electronic storage devices.

✧✧✦✧✧

Death of a Doyenne, Gangubai

Gangubai Hangal died in July 2009 at the ripe old age of ninety-five. With her death, a chapter in Hindustani Classical Music came to an end. I feel compelled to write about her and her music.

Classical music of this country has evolved over the last two thousand years. Though there are structural similarities, the music evolved differently in the north and south of this country. Strangely, some of the giants of Hindustani [North Indian Classical] music originated from a small region in the north of Karnataka, which is in South India. Gangubai came from this part of the country.

Classical music has been derived from many sources, such as tribal folk singing and devotional music. The spontaneity of tribal and devout singers was channeled into a format that grew into an art form over many centuries.

Many schools of music, called *gharanas*, took up certain aspects of the music and specialised, without deviating from the original structure of the *raag* [melody] and *tala* [rhythm]. *Kirana* gharana is one of them, and Gangubai was the outstanding exponent of this gharana's music.

What is it about her music that makes her so special? It is very difficult to define the character of classical music. It has to be felt, and in her music, one could experience the power of Indian classical music. She did not have a great voice, unlike her much-loved daughter Krishna, who died young due to cancer.

Her voice sounded neither male nor female and could even be termed *harsh*. It was not the voice that held you, but the special quality of rendering, which, though well within the structure of the raag, transcended the limits and went beyond, which lovers of classical music came to appreciate.

She was also one of those who refused to compromise. For her, concerts of limited time were an anathema. To elaborate on one raag, one often needs more than an hour, and she would not accept any invitation that was time-bound. She therefore gave fewer performances than others, and it became even fewer after the death of her beloved daughter, Krishna Hangal.

Honours came to her aplenty. There were no fewer than five honorary doctorates conferred on this simple woman from a small town. Though Gangubai remained a simple woman at heart, her music rose to great heights.

She will be missed.

❖❖◆❖

Postscript

What does one gain after reading the stories in this book?

For doctors and those closely associated with the profession, these stories will reveal the richness and the quality of family medicine, a crucial field within healthcare. These may motivate some of them, especially if they are students, to take up this as their career choice. For lay readers, these stories illustrate the importance of the institution of family medicine in safeguarding their health.

There is a trend towards institutional care for ailments which can be managed at home. When 90% of illnesses can be managed at home by competent primary care doctors, and of the remaining 10%, only some 8% need specialist help, and just 2% need hospital care, why is there a need to go to hospitals for each and every sundry complaint? This situation has arisen because of a paucity of family doctors in the community.

The future of family medicine, and that of the whole medical profession, is uncertain. With rapid digitalisation and a headlong jump into Artificial Intelligence, the possibility of robots taking over many aspects of present-day medicine, including family medicine, looms large.

What about human-to-human interaction if this were to happen? One cannot predict.

Until then,

Those of you who have read this book, seek help from your family doctor first and follow their counsel for your health needs. If you do this, *I consider my job done.*

If you do not have a family doctor, it is time to seek one!

A veteran family physician for over five decades,
Dr. [Capt.] B.C. Rao is a graduate of
Bangalore Medical College and is a Diplomate of the
National Board in Family Medicine.

He co-founded the Family Physicians' Association [FPA] of
Bangalore in 1979 with a few of his friends and has been a
dedicated educator and advocate for the field.
He has published several articles in
*Journal of Family Medicine and Primary Care, Indian Journal of
Medical Ethics,* and *The National Medical Journal of India.*

A collection of his insights and experiences, interwoven with
personal biographical threads, are captured in his published memoir:
A Family Physician's Life.

He currently mentors the Karnataka branch of the
AFPI [Academy of Family Physicians of India] and
edits its newsletter/journal.

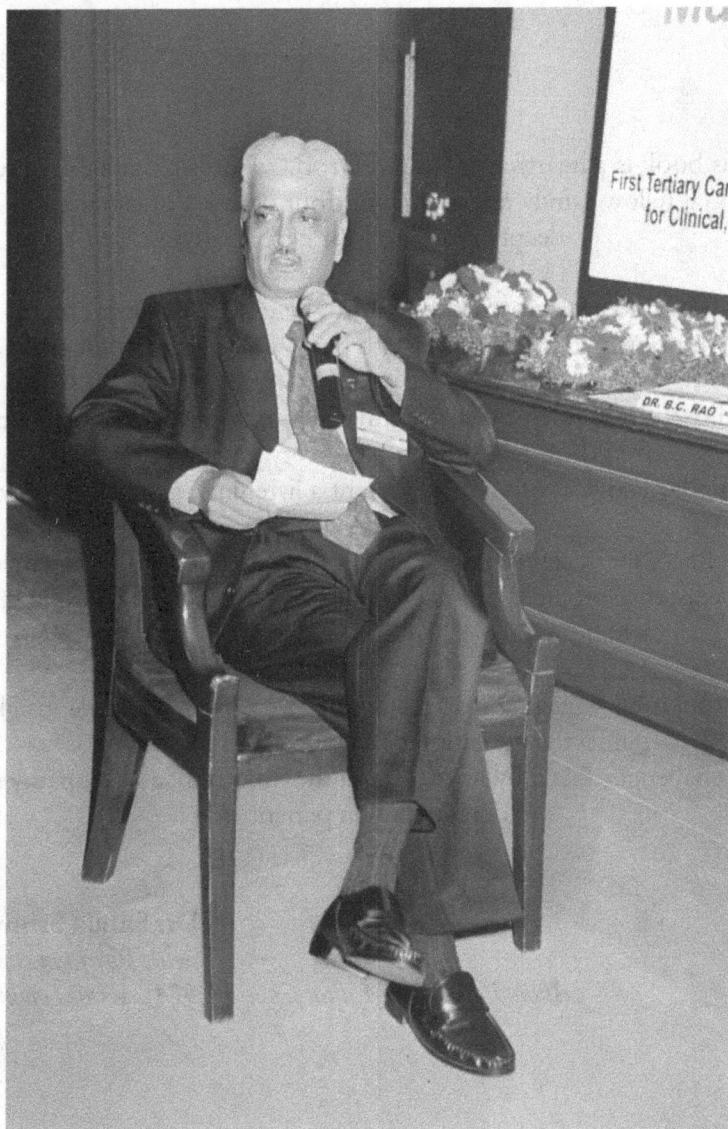

Dr. [Capt.] B.C. Rao

This book is a heartfelt tribute to Dr. B.C. Rao's remarkable career. As a fellow family physician with four decades of experience, I deeply resonate with his narrative.

Dr. Rao's stories vividly capture the unique challenges and responsibilities that came with being a physician in the past.

In those times, doctors wore many hats - physician, therapist, family friend, and confidant. Not every patient required medical advice; often, they sought a listening ear and empathy.

Dr. Rao's work serves as a reminder of the dedication, compassion, and expertise required of being a physician, particularly during an era when the medical landscape was vastly different.

Through his engaging storytelling, Dr. Rao offers valuable insights into the evolution of the medical profession, the challenges faced by doctors, and the importance of empathy and understanding in patient care.

Dr. Sarala Srinivas,
Family Physician (Retd.),
Alumni, Andhra Medical College (1974), Visakhapatnam.

"This unforgettable book is a testament to the transformative power of stories, exploring themes of hope, healing, and the unwavering strength of the human spirit."

— **Arun Felbin,**
Vice President, KEC Transmission & Distribution, Kolkata.

"When a doctor exchanges his stethoscope for a pen, a healing author evolves with a profound and in-depth knowledge of humanity and life, through which a fresh perspective on healthcare emerges…"

— **Rekha Narendra,**
Senior Vice President (Human Resources), RealPage, Hyderabad.

"Half a century of healing unfolds: patient tales, wit, wisdom, and the ethical heart of medicine. This unputdownable book chronicles a veteran physician's remarkable journey."

— **Sreedhara Reddy Mallavarapu,**
Director, Software Engineering, Honeywell.

"The Doctor's journey from stethoscope to pen is nothing but sublime prose which soothes the soul and is a therapeutic balm for the mind."

— **Kamal Narendra,**
President, Rotary Club Of Madras Mid-town.

"The stories and anecdotes conveyed the closeness between a family doctor and his patients, revealing a personal rapport going beyond the clinicality of a doctor-patient relationship into the emotional realm too."

— **Anuja Kolhatkar,**
Academician and Founder, Helixx Insights, Pune.

"This book mirrors Dr. Rao's pragmatic, humorous advice, which we've experienced for more than 25 years; often prescription-free, with playful warnings on antibiotics like 'killing a mosquito with a bazooka!' It is both insightful and empathetic."

— **Swathi Reddy,**
Entrepreneur.

www.ingramcontent.com/pod-product-compliance
Lightning Source LLC
Chambersburg PA
CBHW011158220326
41597CB00028BA/4702